The Complete MRCGP Study Guide

Second Edition

Sarah Gear

General Practitioner
Cheshire

Radcliffe Publishing
Oxford • Seattle

Radcliffe Publishing Ltd
18 Marcham Road
Abingdon
Oxon OX14 1AA
United Kingdom

www.radcliffe-oxford.com
Electronic catalogue and worldwide online ordering facility.

British Library Cataloguing in Publication Data

A catalogue record for this book is available from the British Library.

ISBN-10: 1 85775 780 7
ISBN-13: 978 1 85775 780 4

Typeset by Aarontype Ltd, Easton, Bristol
Printed and bound by TJ International Ltd, Padstow, Cornwall

Contents

About the author

Dr Sarah Gear graduated in 1995 from Manchester Medical School. She undertook SHO posts followed by the GP vocational training scheme at the North Staffordshire Royal Infirmary in Stoke-on-Trent, qualifying as a GP in August 2001 and successfully gaining the MRCGP the same year.

In April 2002, she became a principal at her former training practice in Madeley, near Crewe.

Acknowledgements

From the initial workbook versions to the final format of the second edition was not achieved without the help and encouragement of my friends and colleagues. Both Kate, with our many hours of preparation for the MRCGP together, and James, who didn't mind (too much) the sacrifice of our evenings, have been instrumental in the production of this work. The many courses and study days run by my colleagues have been a necessity in both keeping up to date and putting the works in the journals into a working perspective.

Gillian Nineham and her initial belief in the project, Jamie Etherington for his ongoing support and advice throughout the publication of both editions, and the whole team at Radcliffe for the advice and polite suggestions on how to improve my grammar (which has sometimes left me smiling for days!). Without such dedication I would still be printing off individual workbooks for circulation. Thank you.

Introduction

It is important to establish from the outset that the exam is not about knowing everything. Let's face it, there would be little point in knowing all about the treatment of Indian visceral leishmaniasis for day-to-day general practice. Many studies that influence general practice today were completed years ago. Being able to regurgitate a textbook, hot topics or otherwise, does not mean that you've got the exam cracked. It certainly doesn't make you a better doctor.

The College website (www.rcgp.org.uk) is a must. Even if you have sat the exam before, you must read the rules again – they can change, so don't be caught out.

Part of the groundwork is to speak to as many people as possible about their learning techniques and approach for the MRCGP. You will find that in the majority of cases people will identify a topic ('learning need') and read around it from, say, a textbook. Then they might do a Medline search for current review articles or look in *Clinical Evidence* to check whether there is any new, revolutionary information that might change the way they would tackle the given subject (i.e. the way they practise).

The more enlightened doctors manage to keep up to date with the journals and comics, do their own video analysis and even have a mentor. This would form part of a personal development plan (PDP). Thinking about what you would want to achieve in general practice from early on in your career will mean you can maximise what you get out of your hospital jobs.

To be a medically competent GP you need to be well read (a true generalist) and have an open, sensible approach to acquiring knowledge that will fill in any gaps. You need to be able to work as part of a team (you will be part of the primary healthcare team, not to mention the doctor–patient aspect), and you need to be open to ethical and cultural ideas and beliefs. That's all just for starters!

In this book I have covered the main medical topics that are fundamental to general practice. This is not meant to provide comprehensive coverage of aetiology, pathophysiology, investigations and treatments – quite the opposite. I assume that if you aren't up to speed and need to recap, you will be able to access this information easily. I have incorporated current treatment issues, National Service Frameworks, the latest research, questions, etc. It is all clearly referenced and the issues are not clouded by my personal opinions – the whole point to postgraduate learning is to formulate your own. Having said that, where it seemed important to do so, I have included the opinions of published authors from the journals.

All this is to save you the colossal amount of time that you would otherwise need to prepare for the exam.

Finally, it is important to remember the following.

- You don't need to know everything (you cannot possibly).
- It is easier if what you are learning is topical/relevant.
- It is not how much you know, but how you apply that knowledge, that matters.
- Hot topics form only a small part of the exam, be it MRCGP or summative assessment.
- You generally do not need to quote specific references.

Sarah Gear
May 2006
gear@doctors.org.uk

How to use this book

Probably the worst thing you could do at this stage is to try and plough through from beginning to end – you would never make it, and even if you did, you would be unlikely to remember much of it.

Use the book as a starting point, a guide or for summing up to ensure that you are as well read as you think you are. Flick through and get a handle on the layout and what is included. No doubt there will be parts you know inside out – so don't be tempted to spend too much time here, move on. Scribble comments and questions, highlight text, use Post-it notes or completely deface it if necessary. Do whatever you like, but make sure it works for you.

As you go through the different sections, think not only of possible questions the examiners might set, but also how you would explain the various issues if you had to teach the subject. Write down the questions you come up with and use them for revision.

With regard to the exam-style questions, each part explains what is involved and suggests ways of tackling them (e.g. against the clock, in pairs, etc.). All answers are comprehensive but not exhaustive. As you get used to the techniques and increase your knowledge base, there will be points that you feel are important which I have not included – keep them as part of your answer.

No book will ever cover everything you need to know, but this one encompasses a huge amount. I hope you find it an indispensable guide to both your GP registrar year and the MRCGP.

General practice is a fantastic career, and although the MRCGP is not yet essential, it is a worthwhile exam to work for. You will gain an incredible amount from it if you are willing to put in the time and effort.

Enjoy and good luck!

Part I

Coronary heart disease (CHD)

National Service Framework for CHD

Launched in March 2000 (www.doh.gov.uk/nsf/coronary.htm), this is a follow-on from the White Paper *Saving Lives: our healthier nation*, in which CHD was set out as a priority.

It is a 10-year plan which:

- aims to reduce death from CHD and stroke by 40% by 2010 in people up to 75 years of age
- emphasises the need to provide structured, systematic care.

Since its launch, statin prescribing has doubled.

There are 12 standards, but the following priorities are highlighted:

- smoking cessation advice
- CHD register in primary care
- rapid assessment chest pain clinic
- faster treatment for myocardial infarction, and improved secondary prevention
- more heart operations/revascularisation.

Standards that mainly affect primary care

- Standard 2 – smoking cessation advice.
- Standards 3 and 4 – these cover secondary prevention followed by primary prevention:
  - comprehensive CHD register for audit purposes
  - development of protocols and guidelines (these need to be agreed at practice level, primary care group/trust level and across primary, secondary and tertiary care).
- Standard 11 – heart failure and palliative care for people with CHD – we are responsible for arranging appropriate investigations to confirm diagnosis and then offering appropriate treatment.

Workload issues

These include the following:

- identifying patients and maintaining registers
- regular audit (every 3 months)
- practice time (meetings, clinics, following protocols and guidelines, etc.)
- treating the patient/pharmacology.

Secondary prevention of coronary heart disease in older patients after the national service framework: population based study
BMJ 2006; 332: 144–5

This study looked at men and women with established coronary heart disease at two time points (respectively 817 and 465 in 1998–2001, 857 and 548 in 2003) aged 60–79 years in 1998–2001. They found that statin uptake and the use of combined drug treatment in elderly men and women increased markedly (from 34% to 65% and from 48% to 67% respectively). There was still room for further improvement with beta-blockers and ACE inhibitors.

If we as GPs are to be held accountable (which we will be), then we need adequate staffing with appropriate training.
  Interestingly, *Health Statistics Quarterly* (www.nationalstatistics.gov.uk) gives weight to the argument that GPs do not need government guidance to keep their practice up to date. Prescribing habits had changed appropriately prior to the publication of the National Service Framework (as was seen with angiotensin converting enzyme (ACE) inhibitors in congestive cardiac failure).

Hypertension

This is bread-and-butter general practice, and you must know these guidelines. With a prevalence of around 11%, you would be unlucky not to see this every day of your working life.

British Hypertension Society Guidelines 2004
J Hum Hypertens 2004; 18: 139–85 and *BMJ* 2004; 328: 634–40 (summary)

The British Hypertension Society (BHS) published a 2004 update of previous guidelines (1989, 1993 and 1999). The guidelines state that the main determinant of benefit from blood pressure-lowering drugs is the achieved blood pressure rather than the choice of therapy.

Summary of BHS Guidelines

- Start antihypertensive treatment in patients with:
    - a sustained systolic BP $\geqslant 160$ mmHg
    - a sustained diastolic BP $\geqslant 100$ mmHg.

- Start antihypertensive treatment in diabetic patients who have:
    - systolic BP $\geqslant 140$ mmHg
    - diastolic BP $\geqslant 90$ mmHg.

- Treat borderline blood pressure (140–159/90–99 mmHg) if there is target organ damage, cardiovascular disease, diabetes or a 10-year cardiovascular disease risk $\geqslant 20\%$ (this is equivalent to the CHD risk of around 15%).

- Optimal BP targets in non-diabetics are:
    - systolic BP < 140 mmHg
    - diastolic BP < 85 mmHg.

- The minimum acceptable control for audit purposes is 150/90 mmHg, and for patients with diabetes, chronic renal disease and established cardiovascular disease (CVD) it is 130/80 mmHg.

- Give non-pharmacological advice to all hypertensives (and borderline hypertensives).

- Consider statins to reduce cardiovascular risk in:
  − primary prevention, where the 10-year cardiovascular risk factor is $\geqslant 20\%$
  − secondary prevention, where high blood pressure is complicated by CVD (irrespective of the baseline total cholesterol).

- Optimal cholesterol lowering should reduce the total cholesterol by 25% (or LDL-cholesterol by 30%) or achieve a cholesterol <4.0 mmol/l (or LDL-cholesterol <2.0 mmol/l) − whichever is the greater reduction.

- Consider aspirin (75 mg/day), when the BP is controlled (<150/90 mmHg) in:
  − primary prevention if over 50 years of age with a 10-year CVD risk $\geqslant 20\%$
  − secondary prevention of ischaemic cardiovascular disease.

The guidelines are based on the HOT trial, summarised below.

Hypertension − management of hypertension in adults in primary care NICE August 2004 (www.nice.org.uk)

NICE and the BHS differ mainly in their approach to drug treatments. The BHS suggests that triple therapy would be a combination of an ACE inhibitor (A), calcium-channel blocker (C) and diuretic (D), with beta-blockers being used for patients who do not respond to or who are intolerant of other medication. NICE recommends a thiazide diuretic and a beta-blocker first line, except in those at risk of diabetes.

NICE is reviewing its guidance in light of the ASCOT trial. It is hoped that a definitive guidance might be agreed upon.

Effects of intensive BP lowering and low-dose aspirin in patients with hypertension: principal results of the Hypertension Optimal Treatment (HOT) randomised trial
Lancet 1998; 351: 1755−62

This trial included 18,790 patients in 26 countries (with a follow-up of 3.8 years on average). It looked at outcomes in terms of major cardiovascular events. Felodipine (a calcium-channel antagonist) was the baseline therapy.

The lowest incidence of major cardiovascular events, a 30% reduction, occurred at a mean achieved diastolic blood pressure of 83 mmHg. For diabetes, the lowest incidence was found at a BP of <80 mmHg.

Daily addition of aspirin 75 mg reduced the risk of myocardial infarction by 36% in men, in well-controlled hypertension.

Anglo-Scandinavian Cardiac Outcome Trials – BP-lowering arm (ASCOT-BPLA)
Lancet 2005; 366: 895–906

This trial has attracted a huge amount of attention, as up until this publication no trial had found an antihypertensive regime that was better than a thiazide and beta-blocker combination (for morbidity, mortality and cost-effectiveness).

It was a randomised controlled trial of 19,257 patients (aged 40–79 years) with hypertension and at least three additional risk factors (not including patients who had recently had a myocardial infarction, stroke or angina). The patients were randomised to receive either atenolol (and a thiazide if needed) or amlodipine (and perindopril if needed).

The primary end point (non-fatal myocardial infarction and fatal coronary heart disease) showed no significant difference; however, the amlodipine group found:

- fewer patients developing new-onset diabetes (5.9% vs. 8.3%; HR 0.70, 95% CI 0.63–0.78)

- significantly better outcome in secondary end points – including cardiovascular mortality and strokes.

This issue is not so much with thiazide diuretics as with beta-blockers first line; it is not clear whether or not it is a class effect. At present this trial helps to build on our current knowledge on the cautious use of beta-blockers as first-line therapy.

Cardiovascular protection and blood pressure reduction
Lancet 2001; 358: 1305–6

This meta-analysis of nine drug trials (62,605 patients) showed little difference in the outcome of antihypertensive effects of diuretics, beta-blockers, calcium-channel blockers and ACE inhibitors. The emphasis was on the fact that it is the ultimate blood pressure control that is important.

Major outcomes in high-risk hypertensive patients randomised to ACEI or Ca-channel blockers vs. diuretics: the antihypertensive and lipid-lowering treatment to prevent heart attack trial (ALLHAT Trial)
JAMA 2002; 288: 2981–97

This multicentre randomised controlled trial involving 42,418 patients over 55 years confirmed the above meta-analysis. It was concluded that the most important factor in reducing risk and mortality is reducing the blood pressure, not the actual drug used.

Blood pressure-measuring devices

Most sphygmomanometers in general practice are not serviced and calibrated, which means that GPs may misclassify patients. The need for recalibration has been emphasised by the BHS since 1986.

The Government, following a report by the Medicines and Healthcare Products Regulatory Agency (MHRA) warning that oscillometric devices were often inaccurate, has recommended the following:

- Where mercury devices are used maintain safety procedures, such as spillage kits.

- Do not assume CE-marked oscillometric devices are suitable for diagnosis of hypertension.

- Use alternative devices where oscillometric devices are unsuitable (e.g. arrhythmias).

- Aneuroid devices should be checked regularly.

- The NHS must purchase only devices that meet MHRA standards.

BP Measuring devices: recommendations of the European Society of Hypertension
BMJ **2001; 322:531–6**

This is a rather dry read, emphasising recalibration in accordance with BHS protocols and standards set by the US Association for the Advancement of Medical Instrumentation (AAMI).

Hypertension in the elderly

Half of all people over 60 years have hypertension. Several age-specific studies have provided evidence about treating hypertension in the elderly.

Further learnings from the European Working Party on Hypertension in the Elderly (EWPHE) study: focus on systolic hypertension
Cardiovascular Drug Therapy **1991; 4 Suppl: 1249–51**

In this study of 840 patients aged over 60 years and with BP $>160/90$ mmHg, thiazide vs. placebo produced a significant reduction in cardiovascular mortality and death from myocardial infarction.

Diagnosis and treatment of isolated systolic hypertension in the elderly project: results of a survey four years post-SHEP
Am J Geriatr Cardiol **1997; 6(4):21–36**

In the original 1991 study of 4,736 patients over 60 years and with BP $>160/90$ mmHg, thiazide vs. placebo (could switch to atenolol or reserpine if thiazide was ineffective) caused a reduction in all major cardiovascular events (especially marked in the diabetic subgroup). In the follow-up review it was found that physicians' attitudes and approaches had meant an increased use of ACE inhibitors and calcium-channel blockers in this cohort of people.

MRC and STOP H Trials have both confirmed the above.

BHS guidelines recommend that drug treatment is of proven benefit up to 80 years of age and once started it should be continued. If diagnosed after the age of 80 years, base the decision to treat on the clinical picture; thiazides are the preferred first-line therapy.

Organisational factors in relation to control of blood pressure: an observational study
Br J Gen Pract **2005; 55: 931–7**

Historically, studies have shown that 60–75% of patients with hypertension treated in general practice do not reach blood pressure targets of 150/90 mmHg. This study looked at 560 randomly selected patients (aged 40–79 years) undergoing treatment and found that 49% had adequate control (i.e. half the patients were uncontrolled). This is slightly better than (but in keeping with) previous studies.

Heart failure

Wilson (1997) described heart failure as:

> a complex clinical syndrome characterised by abnormalities in left ventricular function, neurohormonal regulation, exercise intolerance, shortness of breath, fluid retention and reduced longevity.

Heart failure is not a diagnosis, it can include features of impaired left ventricular function or reduced cardiac output seen in a number of conditions. You need to consider causes such as ischaemic heart disease, hypertension, arrhythmias, cardiomyopathy, valvular heart disease, etc., as this will help you deliver the correct management plan. There is poor correlation between symptoms and signs when comparing the echocardiographic findings to degree of impairment.

Heart failure has been targeted by Standard 11 of the National Service Framework, as it is known that we under-diagnose and under-treat heart failure. It highlights the need for correct diagnosis and appropriate investigation.

- Prevalence is 3–20 per 1,000 among the general population.
- Prevalence is 100 per 1,000 if over 65 years of age.
- Afro-Caribbeans over 65 years of age are at 2.5 times greater risk.

Management of chronic heart failure in adults in primary and secondary care
NICE October 2003 (www.nice.org.uk)

This is a comprehensive guide for heart failure in the following areas.

- Diagnosis:
  - a 12-lead ECG and/or BNP* (or NTproBNP*) are recommended. If one or more is found to be abnormal then echocardiography is recommended
  - other recommended tests include chest X-ray, urea and electrolytes, haemoglobin, glucose, thyroid function tests, etc.

---

*BNP = B-type natriuretic peptide; NTproBNP = N-terminal pro-BNP.

- Treatment:
  - ACE inhibitors are recommended for left ventricular systolic dysfunction (LVSD)
  - beta-blockers should be started in LVSD after ACE inhibitors and diuretics, regardless of whether symptoms persist.

- Monitoring:
  - clinical states, including cardiac rhythm, cognitive and nutritional status should be assessed
  - review of medication
  - urea, electrolytes and creatinine.

- Referral and approach to care.

- Supporting patients and carers.

- Anxiety and depression.

- End-of-life issues.

Diagnosis

The European Society of Cardiology's guidelines for diagnosis of heart failure include the following.

- *Essential*: symptoms – shortness of breath, swollen ankles, fatigue and objective evidence of cardiac dysfunction at rest.

- *Non-essential*: response to treatment directed towards heart failure.

Diagnostic accuracy
It is known (Finland report and the ECHOES study) that 60–80% of people with a diagnosis of heart failure may not have consistent features on echocardiography.

Barriers to accurate diagnosis and effective management of heart failure in primary care: qualitative study
BMJ 2003; 326: 196–200

This study identified three reasons why GPs had difficulty in diagnosing and managing heart failure:

1 uncertainty about clinical practice
  - diagnostic process – third heart sound, raised jugular venous pulse (especially in obese patients)
  - availability and use of echocardiography services
  - treatment issues

2 lack of awareness of relevant research evidence

3 influences of individual preferences and local organisational factors.

Despite the lack of diagnostic accuracy there have been some studies that found the diagnosis made by hospital physicians was equally as inaccurate.

If we were to refer everyone for echocardiography the system would be overwhelmed. It has been suggested that we refer patients whose ECG or chest X-ray are abnormal. Interestingly, the National Service Framework stated that open-access echocardiography should be available to all GPs by April 2002.

New York Heart Association (NYHA) grading of dyspnoea or angina

Grade	Criteria
1	Symptoms only occur on severe exertion; almost normal lifestyle possible
2	Symptoms occur on moderate exertion; patients have to avoid certain situations (e.g. carrying shopping up stairs)
3	Symptoms occur on mild exertion; activity is markedly restricted
4	Symptoms occur frequently, even at rest

Natriuretic peptides

Brain natriuretic peptide (BNP and NTproBNP) is found at high levels in patients with impaired left ventricular systolic function (due to increased pressure or volume overload of the myocardium). As yet there are conflicting studies related to practical use, as there is a low positive predictive value (other factors that increase BNP are age, renal failure, drugs such as beta-blockers or ACE inhibitors). A role may develop for its use in helping to determine who to send for echocardiography as well as for monitoring treatment.

Treatment of heart failure

NICE reviewed treatment in its 2003 guidance and the *Drugs and Therapeutics Bulletin* published a review in April 2000.

Diuretics

These are essential for symptomatic management (first-line treatment). Their long-term effect on mortality is not known, and it would be unethical to conduct a randomised controlled trial, given the known benefits of treatment.

- Potassium-sparing diuretics (e.g. amiloride).

- Spironolactone (competitive aldosterone inhibitor).

Both the RALES and the EPHESUS trials have shown improved mortality and morbidity values with treatment.

The effect of spironolactone on aldosterone evaluation study investigators
RALES Trial (Randomised Aldactone Evaluation Study)
NEJM **1999; 341: 709–17**

In this study, 1,663 patients with NYHA grade 4 disease who were already on an ACE inhibitor and a loop diuretic (i.e. severe heart failure) were randomised to either spironolactone 25 mg/day or placebo. Improved mortality (a reduction in the risk of death of 30%) was seen when spironolactone was used to block aldosterone receptors in addition to standard therapy. Hyperkalaemia was uncommon if a low dose (25 mg/day) was used.

ACE inhibitors

Trials have consistently shown prolonged survival, reversal of left ventricular hypertrophy and a reduced need for hospital admission due to left ventricular dysfunction when patients are on ACE inhibitors.

The results of the HOPE Study (Heart Outcomes Prevention Evaluation Study) suggest that everyone with heart failure without contra-indications should be on an ACE inhibitor.

The numbers needed to treat (NNT) quoted in different papers are as follows:

- for 1 year to prevent one death 74 if ACE inhibitors alone are used

- for 1 year to prevent one death 29 if ACE inhibitors plus beta-blocker are used.

An International Survey of the Management of Heart Failure in Primary Care was presented in September 2001. A total of 1,000 GPs were questioned, and it was found that 90% were aware of the benefits of ACE inhibitors, 90% were sending patients for ECGs and 80% were sending patients for chest X-rays. About one-third referred patients for echocardiography (services were thought to be inadequate). Although ACE inhibitors were being used, they were being given at inadequate doses. Only 19% of GPs were starting treatment with beta-blockers, and only 30% of patients under the age of 70 years with heart failure were receiving them.

Reassuringly, as GPs, our knowledge of heart failure is quite high and we are starting to have success with ACE inhibitors, but we need to promote beta-blockers in a similar way.

Listed below are brief summaries of the relevant trials.

- CONSENSUS I 1987 (Co-operative North Scandinavian Enalapril Study): this study showed decreased mortality (with 20 mg enalapril bd) after a follow-up period of 1 year in patients with severe heart failure (NYHA grade 4).

- SOLVD 1991 (Study of Left Ventricular Dysfunction): this study showed benefits with enalapril 10 mg bd (with a follow-up period of 4 years). SOLVD-P confirmed that progression of the disease was slowed even if the patient was asymptomatic.

The following trials support the use of ACE inhibitors after myocardial infarction.

- SAVE 1992 (Survival and Ventricular Enlargement Trial): this found that long-term administration of captopril reduced the risk of fatal and non-fatal stroke by 21% (95% CI 5–35).

- AIRE 1993 (Acute Infarction Ramipril Efficacy Study): ramipril was given to 1,014 patients (out of 2,006 for randomisation) following an acute myocardial infarction.

There was an observed 27% risk reduction of all causes of mortality in the ramipril group (95% CI 11–40).

- TRACE 1995 (Trandalopril Cardiac Evaluation Study): trandalopril was seen to reduce mortality and progression to heart failure (1,749 patients were randomly assigned to receive trandalopril). The benefit was seen as early as 30 days into the treatment.

Beta-blockers
Beta-blockers are thought to work by their effects on the renin–angiotensin system and anti-arrhythmic properties in all degrees of heart failure. Over 20 randomised controlled trials involving 20,000 patients have been conducted. They have found that the number needed to treat (NNT) is 29 if beta-blockers and ACE inhibitors are both used (to prevent one death over 1 year).

Beta-blockers are only indicated in moderate heart failure secondary to ischaemia (confirmed by echocardiography). They should be started slowly and titrated. Below is a brief summary of the main trials.

- CIBIS (Cardiac Insufficiency Bisoprolol Study): the results were not significant but the trend was towards improvement in survival.

- CIBIS II: bisoprolol was superior to placebo for mortality and morbidity (32%). The trial was stopped early because the results were so dramatic.

- CAPRICORN: this study found that carvedilol was superior to placebo for mortality and morbidity following myocardial infarction. The trial was stopped early.

- COPERNICUS: this study found that carvedilol improved mortality even in severe heart failure.

- SENIORS: nebivolol improved mortality in elderly patients. However, patients over 75 years of age gained less benefit.

Angiotensin II receptor antagonists
The following randomised controlled trials have found positive results.

- ELITE (Evaluation of Losartan in the Elderly): this tolerability study of losartan vs. captopril in patients over 65 years of age suggested there was a benefit to patients who could not tolerate ACE inhibitors.

- ELITE II: losartan proved not to be superior to captopril with regard to survival. There was a confirmed better tolerability in this trial of 3,152 patients.

- Val-HeFT: in this trial of 366 patients who were not on ACE inhibitors, valsartan was used as an additional treatment. There was a significant reduction in all causes of mortality (by up to 33% if patients had not already been receiving an ACE inhibitor).

- CHARM: in this study candesartan was used (double-blind, randomised controlled trial of 7,599 patients), and it was found that good adherence to medication was associated with a 15% lower risk of death ($p = 0.011$).

- VALIANT: this study randomised 14,703 patients to receive captopril, valsartan or both. It found that valsartan was as effective as an ACE inhibitor in patients with left ventricular systolic dysfunction after myocardial infarction (i.e. the outcomes were not statistically significantly different between the two groups).

Digoxin

It is known that digoxin prevents clinical worsening of heart failure and gives improvement of symptoms. The two main trials that found this to be the case were:

- RADIANCE (Randomised Assessment of Digoxin on Inhibitors of ACE) and

- PROVED study (Prospective Randomised Study of Ventricular Failure and the Efficacy of Digoxin).

One trial has found no reduction in mortality:

- DIG (Digoxin Investigators Group): this trial of 6,800 patients with heart failure but no atrial fibrillation found no decrease in mortality, but there was a reported symptomatic improvement in patients.

Vasodilators

- V-HeFT I nd II: Hydralazine and isosorbide dinitrate vs. placebo (I) or Enalapril (II); there was improved mortality with these drugs, which was not as good as the improvement seen with enalapril (i.e. this is an alternative in renal failure patients).

Multidisciplinary approaches to nutrition, patient counselling and education

There have been six randomised controlled trials of highly selected patients looking at the multidisciplinary approach to care. These showed reduced hospital admission rates, better education and improved quality of life.

Randomised controlled trial of specialist nurse intervention in heart failure
BMJ 2001; 323: 715–18

This trial showed that home-based intervention from nurses can reduce admissions. This is thought to be due to education, treatment and regular contact. This is interesting in light of the recent community matron posts that have been introduced.

Exercise and heart failure

A great deal of attention is given to exercise therapy, across all chronic disease groups, looking at improvement in quality of life, exercise tolerance and, hopefully, reduced morbidity and mortality. The British Heart Foundation has produced several factsheets around exercise (www.bhf.org.uk/factfiles). The current advice (for fit, healthy people) is 30 minutes of exercise a day. In people with limitations, exercise should be within these limitations.

Exercise training meta-analysis of trials in patients with chronic heart failure (ExTraMATCH Collaboration)
BMJ 2004; 328: 189–92

Meta-analysis of randomised controlled trials gives no evidence that properly supervised medical training programmes for patients with heart failure are dangerous. There is clear evidence of an overall reduction in mortality.

Under-treatment in heart failure

Despite all the evidence, we are all aware of polypharmacy and see first hand the iatrogenic problems that can arise as a result of the care we offer when treating people in line with national guidelines. This is highlighted in the following publication.

Public awareness of heart failure in Europe: first results from SHAPE
Eur Heart J 2005; 26(22): 2413–21

This first part of the SHAPE study showed that of the 7,958 lay people completing the survey, only 3% could correctly identify heart failure from a description of typical signs and symptoms. Part of the study design included a survey of 378 GPs in the UK (due to be published in 2006), which found that only 20% regularly prescribed beta-blockers, 36% started heart failure treatment either alone or in combination with a diuretic (the lowest of any country in the study), and that 75% were diagnosing heart failure by signs and symptoms alone.

Cardiovascular disease: lipids and statins

Around 55% of the UK population have a total cholesterol concentration of >5.5 mmol/l, in 25% it is >6.5 mmol/l and in 5% it is >7.8 mmol/l.

Serum cholesterol levels can vary by up to 20% through the course of the day (i.e. the sample needs to be taken while the patient is fasting).

Primary prevention evidence

- AF/TexCAPS (Air Force/Texas Coronary Atherosclerosis Prevention Study): primary prevention of placebo vs. lotorvostatin 20–40 mg was studied in 5,608 middle-aged males and 997 females, with a 7-year follow-up. There was a 34% decrease in new events, this became evident after 6 months of treatment.

- WOSCOPS (West of Scotland Coronary Prevention Study): primary prevention was studied in high-risk male patients. There was a 22% decrease in mortality and a 25% decrease in coronary events.

- ASCOT (Anglo-Scandinavian Cardiac Outcomes Trial): this trial looked at the effect of adding atorvastatin to antihypertensive treatment in patients with a normal cholesterol level. It found a 30% reduction in myocardial infarction and stroke. The trial was stopped 2 years early and there are huge financial implications for the NHS.

Treatment in primary prevention is difficult despite the availability of risk assessment tools, especially when you consider potential cost. Diet and secondary causes should always be looked at in the first instance. Treatment is advised (BHS and NICE) if the 10-year cardiovascular risk is $\geqslant 20\%$; if the 10-year risk is 10–20%, you need to take local advice in terms of resources, although patients would benefit from treatment, as they are at a moderately high risk of developing cardiovascular problems. The number needed to treat (to prevent one death over 5 years) is 69.

Secondary prevention evidence

- 4S Study (Scandinavian Simvastatin Survival Study): in this triple-blind Scandinavian study (94 centres) of 4,444 patients aged 35–70 years (81.4% of whom were male) with coronary heart disease (angina or myocardial infarction), only 37% were on aspirin, and 57% were on beta-blockers. Simvastatin 20 mg vs. placebo (with a follow-up of 5.4 years) decreased the number of coronary events (42% reduction in mortality; relative risk 0.58; CI 0.46–0.73) and cardiovascular mortality (35%; relative risk 0.65; CI 0.52–0.8).

- LIPID (Long-Term Intervention with Pravastatin in IHD): in this study, 9,000 patients with ischaemic heart disease were randomised to either placebo or pravastatin. There was a 25% decrease in mortality, cardiac events and procedures (6-year follow-up). A trial follow-up in 2002 reinforced the initial findings.

- CARE (Cholesterol and Recurrent Events Trial): post-myocardial infarction patients were treated with pravastatin vs. placebo (with a 5-year follow-up). There was a 22% decrease in mortality, 33% decrease in CHD and 20–31% decrease in stroke.

MRC/BHF Heart Protection Study 2002
This randomised trial (20,536 patients, including 2,000 who were at increased risk of cardiovascular disease and 3,000 with diabetes but no history of cardiovascular disease) of simvastatin vs. antioxidant supplementation (vitamin E, C and beta-carotene) found randomisation to vitamins had no effect on vascular (or other) disease, but appeared safe. Simvastatin 40 mg (as compared to placebo), despite 15% stopping therapy because of side effects, found a 14% reduction in all causes of mortality ($p < 0.001$). It also found a 17% reduction in vascular deaths ($p < 0.0001$), with no significant effect on non-vascular deaths.

Statin treatment should be offered to all patients with atherosclerotic disease (with lifestyle advice) to reduce cholesterol to <5 mmol/l (this will become 4 mmol/l) or by 30%, whichever is greater. The number needed to treat to prevent one death over 5 years is 16.

Randomised trials of secondary prevention programmes in CHD: systematic review
BMJ 2001; 323: 957–62

A total of 12 secondary prevention programmes (including 9,803 patients with coronary heart disease) conclude that disease management programmes improve process of care, reduce admissions and enhance quality of life. Disease management programmes should include patient education, practice guidelines, appropriate consultations, supplies of drugs and ancillary services.

Ezetimibe

This is a new cholesterol-lowering drug option. It works as a selective inhibitor of intestinal cholesterol absorption and can be used in addition to a statin to achieve the cholesterol target (once statin is at the maximum dose, or if a statin is not tolerated). There are limited data so far.

Role of plant stanols

A low-fat, high-fibre diet with five portions of fruit and vegetables (although we understand that more is probably needed) has been advocated for many years. Plant stanols are naturally occurring but have come to our attention with the launch in the supermarkets of Benecol and Flora Pro-active (1 teaspoon a day is the maximum needed for cholesterol-lowering effects).

Plant stanol and stanol margarines and health
BMJ 2000; 320: 861–4

This meta-analysis of all randomised controlled trials showed that a daily intake of 2 g of plant stanols resulted in a 9–14% reduction in LDL-cholesterol levels.

Cardiovascular disease and antiplatelets

Aspirin has been advised for primary and secondary prevention of cardiovascular disease in high-risk patients for many years. Although not completely supported by evidence, healthy patients use it for many reasons, including to reduce the risk of bowel cancer and Alzheimer's disease.

Aspirin works by blocking cyclo-oxygenase, which then has the knock-on effect of reducing platelet aggregation (through reduction in thromboxaneA2 and prostocycline). Clopidogrel inhibits platelet aggregation by interacting with the platelet ADP receptor. The *MeRec Bulletin* July 2005 (volume 15) gave an excellent overview of options and recommendations for the use of antiplatelets in primary and secondary prevention. It can be summarised as follows.

- Primary prevention
  - low-dose aspirin (75 mg/day) should be considered in all patients over 50 years with a 10-year cardiovascular risk of $\geqslant 20\%$
  - clopidogrel and MR-dipyridamole are not indicated or licensed for primary prevention.
- Secondary prevention
  - low-dose aspirin (75 mg/day) is recommended for indefinite use following a myocardial infarction and in people with symptomatic peripheral arterial disease
  - MR-dipyridamole (200 mg twice daily) plus aspirin (75 mg/day) is recommended for a period of 2 years after an ischaemic stroke or transient ischaemic attack (TIA), from the most recent event

- clopidogrel (75 mg/day) is a suitable alternative to aspirin (or aspirin plus dipyridamole post-stroke) where aspirin is not tolerated (even with a proton-pump inhibitor) or contra-indicated
- clopidogrel (75 mg/day) plus aspirin (75 mg/day) for a period of 12 months should be considered in patients with a non-ST-segment-elevation acute coronary syndrome who are at moderate to high risk of a further myocardial infarction or death. Thereafter treatment should revert to aspirin (75 mg/day).

The polypill

It was proposed by Wald and Law, in 2003, that the polypill would be a medication containing six ingredients: a statin, aspirin, folic acid and three antihypertensives (all at half strength). Initial thoughts were that it should be given to everyone over the age of 55 years (with or without existing cardiovascular disease) without screening, the aim being to reduce the risk of ischaemic heart disease events by up to 88% and stroke by up to 80%. This would be achieved by reducing four risk factors: blood pressure, platelet function, lipid and homocysteine concentrations.

The polypill and cardiovascular disease
BMJ 2005; 330: 1035–6 (Editorial)

This considers that the polypill, based on the available evidence, may be appropriate for secondary prevention but not for primary prevention (due to its non-specific scatter-shot approach).

Cardiovascular disease risk assessments

Individuals are at increased risk of developing CVD if they are smokers, hypertensive, have dyslipidaemias or diabetes mellitus. It is also known that obesity, increased waist:hip ratio and increased alcohol consumption, family history and ethnicity all increase an individual's risk. Preventing CVD can be argued to be one of the most important tasks for GPs.

Absolute risk is the probability of developing CHD (non-fatal myocardial infarction or coronary death) over a defined period of time, and can be estimated using risk assessment charts. These help us to explain risks to the patient, which in turn empowers them to make informed choices on available options. The information from the charts should not replace clinical judgement.

Most risk assessment tools are based on complex mathematics from the Framingham studies, although they are now relatively simple to use. They are for use in *primary prevention*. They are not for use in patients who have existing diseases which already put them at high risk, such as CHD, stroke, atherosclerotic disease, familial hypercholesterolaemia, inherited dyslipidaemia or renal dysfunction (including diabetic nephropathy).

The original Framingham study (named after a town in Massachusetts) was published in 1971, having looked for over 14 years at 2,282 men and 2,845 women, their lipid profiles and CHD risks. Since then a multitude of spin-off studies relating to CHD have been published. The main concerns surrounding the use of Framingham models is that there is no consideration of ethnicity, family history or socioeconomic groupings. For this reason, NICE is considering a review of all risk assessment charts currently used.

The accuracy of the Framingham risk-score in different socioeconomic groups: a prospective study
Br J Gen Pract 2005; 55: 838–845

This study looked at 12,304 men and women with complete risk-factor information and found that there was a relative underestimation of cardiovascular risk (by up to 48%; 95% CI 0.48–0.56) for manual participants, compared to 31% in non-manual. It concluded that the Framingham study underestimated risk in a poor socioeconomic cohort (an area not previously documented).

Joint British Societies coronary risk prediction chart

This chart was produced by British Cardiac, Hypertension, Hyperlipidaemia and Diabetic Associations. It distinguishes between diabetics and non-diabetics, men and women, and smokers and non-smokers. The graphs then depend on systolic blood pressure, total cholesterol : HDL cholesterol ratio and also a person's age.

It sounds complicated, but it is simple to use and can be found in the *British National Formulary* and *MIMS*.

New Zealand tables

These look at the 5-year risk and include the number needed to treat. They are not in regular use in the UK.

Sheffield tables

These look at the 10-year risk and break the estimates down into 15% and 30% risks.

SCORE

This is a project based on the meta-analysis of 12 studies in Europe (involving 250,000 people), as it is thought that the risk assessment tables based on Framingham overestimated the CHD risk in certain subgroups. Individual risk charts will be tailor-made for a specific population.

Problems with tables

These risk assessment tables have all been valuable. They have given us a place to start ongoing evaluations and have helped us work out levels of treatment. However, no system is perfect. Some of the main concerns with the use of risk assessment tables are listed below.

- Tables usually calculate a 10-year risk and this becomes inaccurate with blood pressure and life style changes over time, so you need to reassess periodically.

- They can be time-consuming to include opportunistically in a consultation (despite IT facilities).

- They do not always take into account ethnicity (which can increase the risk by around 1.5).

- They underestimate the risk if there is a strong family history of CHD below 65 years of age, or hyperlipidaemia (in these cases it is thought you need to increase the risk estimate by a factor of 1.5).

Atrial fibrillation (AF)

AF is the most common tachydysrhythmia diagnosed on ECG. It is important to diagnose, as it may be the first sign of heart disease and is an important risk factor for strokes. There is no known cause in 20–30% of cases. However, the majority of cases are associated with hypertension or structural valvular disease.

The prevalence of AF is 1.5% up to 60 years of age, increasing to 8% at 90 years of age. The annual risk of stroke increases from 6.7% in the 50–59-year age band to around 36% in the 80–89-year band.

Warfarin or not?

Many trials have shown that warfarin is superior to aspirin (for both primary and secondary prevention), reducing thromboembolism in non-rheumatic AF by up to 68% (compared with 28%). However, these studies are generally based on patients in secondary care with higher risks, and the selected/excluded patient groups have been quite strict and then well monitored. Most of the studies compared either aspirin or warfarin with placebo, not with each other.

Anticoagulants vs. antiplatelet therapy for preventing stroke in patients with non-rheumatic AF and a history of stroke or TIA
Cochrane Database **2004; 4: CD000187**

The two trials identified were the European Atrial Fibrillation Trial (455 patients received either anticoagulant or aspirin 300 mg/day) and the Studio Italiano Fibrillazione Atriale trial (916 patients randomised to either anticoagulants or indobrufen). After a period of 1 year the combined results showed that anticoagulants were significantly more effective than antiplatelets at preventing all vascular events (OR 0.67; 95% CI 0.50–0.91), and for preventing recurrent stroke (OR 0.49; 95% CI 0.33–0.72). Although major extracranial bleeding occurred more frequently in the anticoagulation group (OR 5.16; 95% CI 2.08–12.83) the absolute difference was small (2.8% per year vs. 0.9% per year – this was worse in the EAFT).

Primary prevention of arterial thromboembolism in non-rheumatic AF in primary care: RCT comparing two intensity coumarin with aspirin
BMJ **1999; 319: 958–64**

In this primary care study of 729 patients over 60 years of age, neither low nor standard intensity anticoagulation was found to be better than aspirin.

Meta-analysis of anti-coagulation/aspirin in non-rheumatic AF: 5 RCT from the past 12 years
BMJ 2001; 322: 321–6

This study found no significant difference in cardiovascular events, although there was a higher risk of bleeds in the warfarin group. Needless to say, certain people are disputing this review which, in itself, underlines the continued rumblings of a lack of consensus.

Co-morbidity associated with atrial fibrillation: a general practice-based study
Br J Gen Pract 2001; 51: 884–90

This recent UK study showed that up to 60% of patients with AF have contraindications for either warfarin or aspirin. When deciding on appropriate treatment in the 40% of patients who are eligible, it is important to discuss the risks vs. the benefits.

Screening

Opportunistic screening is currently being considered as an option. Almost without realising, we selectively screen patients with every blood pressure we take, pulse we feel, heart we listen to and ECG we perform. The study below looked at formalising the process.

A randomised controlled trial and cost-effectiveness study of systematic screening (targeted and total population screening) vs. routine practice for detection of atrial fibrillation in people aged 65 and over. The SAFE study
Health Technol Assess 2005; 9(40): iii–iv, ix–x, 1–74

This study found that opportunistic screening was the most cost-effective method (243 patients in this arm yielded 31 new cases, an incidence of 0.69% in the 12 months of the study) for detection of AF in people aged 65 years and over.

Cardiovascular disease – miscellaneous issues

Cardiac rehabilitation

The aim is to restore the patient to the best possible function after acute coronary syndrome and minimise the risk of recurrence.

British Heart Foundation Factfile 09/2000

Cardiac rehabilitation improves risk, morbidity, mortality and psychosocial outcome. However, it needs to be an individual programme rather than prescriptive, and must have a multidisciplinary approach. Several studies have shown that the programmes are cost-effective (both medically and socially).

The National Service Framework for CHD recommends cardiac rehabilitation as part of secondary prevention within the NHS trust.

An overview of randomised clinical trials of rehabilitation with exercise after MI
Circulation **1989; 80: 234–44**

This showed a reduction in cardiac mortality of 20–25%.

Homocysteine

Homocysteine is an amino acid that stimulates platelet aggregation and thrombus formation (hence atherosclerosis). It is produced as a breakdown product of the animal protein we digest (methionine). The use of folic acid is being considered, and the Government is currently looking into adding folate to flour as a general public health measure.

The current main points are as follows.

- In 2002, the British Cardiac Society presented research showing that elevated homocysteine levels (>12 mmol/l) doubled the risk of a second coronary event.

- High homocysteine levels in the general population are mainly due to insufficient folate and vitamin B concentrations (hence the role of folic acid in the polypill).

- There is not enough evidence to recommend levels as part of the routine CHD risk assessment.

- Guidelines from the International Atherosclerosis Society recommend screening in high-risk patients (not agreed by National Screening Committee). If the levels are checked and found to be raised, treatment with diet or 400 μg folic acid should be initiated and the test repeated after 3 months. If still raised, higher doses of folate, vitamin B6 and vitamin B12 are advocated.

Meta-analysis of MTHFR 677 C → T polymorphism and coronary heart disease: does totality of evidence support causal role for homocysteine and preventative potential of folate?
BMJ **2005; 331: 1053–6**

In this study 26,000 cases and 31,183 controls were included. They found that there was no strong evidence to support an association of the polymorphism and CHD. This casts doubt on the role of folic acid in the prevention of cardiovascular disease.

C-reactive protein (CRP)

A CRP concentration >3 mg/l may indicate the need for intensive treatment to reduce cardiovascular risk. US guidelines suggest case selection and use for patients with a 10-year CHD risk of 10–20%.

Omega-3 fatty acids

It has been known since the 1970s that omega-3 fish oils protect against CHD. The mechanism of action is not fully understood. GISSI 1999 found an absolute risk reduction of 2% (NNT 50).

Risk and benefits of omega-3 fats for mortality, cardiovascular disease, and cancer: systematic review
BMJ 2006; 332: 752–5

This review looked at 48 RCTs (36,913 participants) and 41 cohort studies. The pooled data showed no strong evidence of reduced risk of mortality (relative risk 0.87, 95% CI 0.73–1.03) or combined cardiovascular events (0.95, 0.82–1.12) in people taking additional omega-3 fats.

Nitric oxide

Nitric oxide has been looked at for many years to try and understand its role in endothelial function and repair. In 2005, the first dietary supplement was launched, advocating its use as a primary preventative measure.

Smoking cessation

- Smoking is the number-one preventable cause of ill health (120,000 deaths/year).

- One in four adults in the UK smoke (13 million in total).

- The cost to the NHS is £1,500 million/year.

- 70% of smokers want to stop (National Statistics 2000).

- Smoking cessation by someone with angina may decrease their chances of having a myocardial infarction by up to 50%.

- Smoking data account for 87 of the quality indicator points in the GMS contract (2004).

1998 White Paper *Smoking Kills*

In this framework for the NHS on smoking cessation, funding was initially only guaranteed in New Health Action Zones before being rolled out nationally.
It was recommended that practitioners should:

- assess smoking 'at every opportunity'!

- advise patients to stop smoking

- provide accurate information

- recommend nicotine replacement therapy (NRT)

- refer patients to specialist services as necessary

- follow up patients.

February 2000 Royal College of Physicians initiative on 'Nicotine Addiction in Britain'

- Government should provide access to evidence-based smoking cessation service.

- NRT is effective and should be available by NHS prescription.

- It recommended that GPs give brief advice at least once a year, and if there is a positive response they should refer to a smoking cessation clinic.

Intervention	Success rate at 1 year
Brief opportunistic advice from GP	2%
Face-to-face behavioural support from specialist	7%
Nicotine gum	5%
Zyban (300 mg/day)	9%
Behavioural support in clinic with NRT or Zyban	13–19%

A summary of a recent evaluation of these services was circulated in *CMO Update* (Summer 2005) and found the following.

- Inequalities – success rates are lower among disadvantaged groups.

- Reaching priority groups – there were innovative schemes but also tensions between the need to reach priority groups and achieving quit targets.

- Long-term quit rates – around 15% of people who quit through the services were not smoking at 12 months (compared to 3–4% using willpower alone).

- Service characteristics – better success was seen in models where interventions were used for longer periods of time.

- Cost-effectiveness – it is estimated that the cost per quality-adjusted life year saved was £230–2,700.

Coronary Heart Disease National Service Framework March 2000

- NHS and partner agencies should contribute to a reduction in the prevalence of smoking in the local population.

- Advice about how to stop smoking, including the use of NRT, is highlighted as a high priority in people with diagnosed CHD or other occlusive arterial disease.

- In secondary prevention, annual clinical audit should look at recorded smoking status and, for smokers, the delivery of (or referral for) appropriate advice.

Monitoring Trends and Determinants in Cardiovascular Disease (MONICA) *Lancet* 2000; 355: 668–9

This epidemiological WHO study monitored 100,000 men and women aged 35–64 years from 21 countries over a period of 10 years. The most effective intervention for reducing CHD was stopping smoking (50% risk reduction over 2 years).

Smoking Cessation Action in Primary Care Taskforce (SCAPE), launched in September 2001

- The aim of this initiative was to encourage GPs and practice nurses to maintain the impetus of smoking cessation services.
- It suggests the 30-second approach:
  - do you smoke?
  - would you like to stop?
  - would you like my help with stopping?
- The aim is to catch people at the right point of the cycle of change to help them engage with services.
- A major concern of GPs (in a survey published by SCAPE in May 2001) is workload implications.
- With regard to smoking cessation, 93% of GPs thought it was 'the best thing you could do for their health'.
- Around 91% of GPs put off advising patients to stop because of time pressures.

There have been a lot of published papers looking at ways to encourage patients to stop smoking (including several Cochrane reviews), some are outlined below.

Predictors of long-term outcome of a smoking cessation programme in primary care
Br J Gen Pract **2003; 53: 101–7**

This study showed that the probability of smoking cessation can be predicted. Willingness to participate, increasing age and previous attempts to stop were all positive predictors.

Should smoking cessation cost a packet?
Br J Gen Pract **1999; 49: 127–8**

This does not support the view that free NRT gives better results than if it was bought by the patient.

Mortality among never-smokers living with smokers: two cohort studies 1981–4 and 1996–9
BMJ **2004; 328: 988–9**

This New Zealand study followed two cohorts for 3 years, looking at mortality. They found that in adults who had never smoked, but who had exposure to second-hand smoke in the home, there was an increased mortality – around 15% compared to never-smokers who lived in a smoke-free environment.

NICE 2002 guidelines on smoking cessation treatments (www.nice.org.uk)

- NRT and bupropion are recommended for smokers who want to quit.
- They should only be prescribed if a quit date has been set.

- The initial prescription should ideally last for 2 weeks beyond the quit date and only be continued if the patient is still trying to quit.

- If patients do not stop, another course should not be prescribed for 6 months.

Bupropion is known to lower the seizure threshold so should not be prescribed with a number of other drugs, e.g. antidepressants, antipsychotics, tramadol, theophyllines (check your *British National Formulary*). Similarly, it should not be prescribed to people at risk of seizures or people with diabetes (risk of hypoglycaemia).

Gastrointestinal tract

Dyspepsia

This is defined as 'chronic or recurrent pain or discomfort centred in the upper abdomen'. It is a symptom, not a diagnosis.

Epidemiology of upper dyspepsia in a random population
Scand J Gastroenterol **1994; 29: 1–6**

This is one of many studies to come out of Denmark which found that:

- 13–47% of people have dyspepsia (25% of whom consult their GP, most are endoscopy negative)

- 7% of patients have daily symptoms.

There is a huge amount of literature published on gastro-oesophageal reflux, *Helicobacter pylori*, ulcer and non-ulcer dyspepsia. I suggest the following references for the most up-to-date information:

- NICE Dyspepsia August 2004

- Guidelines – summarising guidelines for primary care (www.eguidelines.co.uk)

- *Clinical Evidence* at www.clinicalevidence.com

Management of dyspepsia in adults in primary care, NICE 2004

The following have been identified as priorities:

- referral for endoscopy
- interventions for uninvestigated dyspepsia
- interventions for gastro-oesophageal reflux disease (GORD)
- interventions for peptic ulcer disease
- interventions for non-ulcer dyspepsia

- reviewing patient care

- *Helicobacter pylori* testing and eradication.

An important part of our initial assessment in primary care is determining if there are any ALARM features (**A**naemia, weight **L**oss, **A**norexia, **R**efractory problems, **M**elaena or swallowing problems) or an acute gastrointestinal bleed that warrants urgent investigation.

Helicobacter pylori

H. pylori is a Gram-negative bacterium that colonises the stomach. It seems to have an aetiological role in gastric and duodenal ulceration, gastric lymphoma, gastric cancer and colorectal adenoma (*J Gastroenterology* 2005; 4099: 887–93). Its exact role in these conditions (and CHD) is unclear.

It affects 20% of people under 40 years of age and 50% of people over 60 years. Reinfection in adults is rare (<1% per year), so eradication is almost curative.

RCT of effects of *Helicobacter pylori* infection and its eradication on heartburn and gastro-oesophageal reflux: Bristol Helicobacter Project
BMJ 2004; 328: 1417

This is the most recent study – 1,558 *H. pylori*-positive people with and without gastro-oesophageal reflux disease showed no difference between eradication treatment and placebo after 2 years. The eradication treatment was neither beneficial nor harmful.

There is still no real conclusion as to whether to eradicate the bacterium from *H. pylori*-positive individuals who have non-ulcer dyspepsia.

Management

In cases of confirmed ulcers, eradication speeds healing and reduces recurrence (NNT = 2). This is not the case in GORD (NNT = 17). Most guidelines suggest that it is not necessary to test for *H. pylori* if there is a known duodenal ulcer, but to treat empirically and investigate if ALARM symptoms occur or they do not improve.

A triple regimen is more successful than the double. There is no difference between the different triple regimens, and 1 week of treatment is as successful as 2 weeks.

Long-term treatment with NSAIDs

Relative contribution of mucosal injury and *H. pylori* in the development of gastrointestinal lesions in patients taking NSAIDs
Gut 2002; 51(3): 329–35

This Swiss study recently advocated a test-and-treat policy for people who require long-term NSAIDs. The randomised controlled trial found that if *H. pylori*-positive patients had eradication therapy while taking NSAIDs, there was a 1% incidence of ulcer. This increased to 6% in those who were untreated.

Non-invasive tests for *H. pylori*

- *Serology*: this does not distinguish between old and active infection (IgG antibodies can remain in the circulation for up to 9 months after eradication), i.e. 50% of positives could be false positives. At present this is a suboptimal test and not recommended. Its sensitivity is 60–85%, and its specificity is 80%, depending on which paper you read.

- *Urea breath test*: urea is hydrolysed by *H. pylori* urease to carbon dioxide and ammonia. The specificity and sensitivity are 95%, and this is thought to be the best test at present. It is easy to use in primary care (but does still have to be sent to the lab for analysis). It should not be used while the patient is taking antacids/proton-pump inhibitors because this causes false-negative results in some cases. The test becomes negative once *H. pylori* is eradicated. It is more expensive than serology but reduces the need for endoscopy, so is more cost-effective in the long run.

- *Stool antigen detection test*: this is usually a monoclonal test (polyclonal tests are less sensitive). The specificity and sensitivity are up to 95%, and you now need only a pea-sized piece of stool. It is not known whether positive tests should ultimately lead to endoscopy to look for secondary pathology. Stool antigen tests should not be performed within 2 weeks of taking proton-pump inhibitors or antibiotics.

Does the test-and-treat strategy work in primary healthcare for management of uninvestigated dyspepsia? A prospective 2-year follow-up study of 1,552 patients
Scand J Gastroenterol **2004; 39(40): 327–35**

Applied in real life, the test-and-treat strategy failed to reduce the number of endoscopies, but significantly reduced peptic ulcer disease and improved dyspeptic symptoms and quality of life.

Invasive test/endoscopy

- *Histology*: has a sensitivity and specificity of >90%. Although it is more invasive and expensive, it is preferable to empirical treatment. It decreases drug consumption, the number of visits to the doctor and sick leave for 2 years after endoscopy compared with the year before, and patients are generally more satisfied with the treatment. The symptomatic outcome (endoscopy vs empirical treatment) is similar in the two groups.

Colorectal cancer

- Colorectal cancer is the second most common cancer in the UK.

- It kills around 16,000 people per year in the UK.

- 5% of people with bowel cancer have more than one cancer.

- 85% of colorectal cancers occur in people over 60 years of age.

Colorectal cancer screening in the UK
Gut 2000; 46: 746–8

Around 90% of cases are diet-related (high fat and meat intake) and 10% are genetic.

Role of the GP

- Identify high-risk patients – early detection improves the 5-year survival.

- Provide detailed counselling and information about causes of colorectal cancer.

- Promote lifestyle issues that may prevent colorectal cancer (eat five portions of fruit and vegetables a day, take 30 minutes of brisk exercise daily, stop smoking and maintain a BMI 18.5–25 kg/m^2 throughout life).

Role of NSAIDs

The use of aspirin as a chemoprotective agent is not yet advocated for the general population. There has been only one randomised controlled trial, with a 5-year follow-up, which showed no benefit. It was postulated that the follow-up was too short and 10–20 years would be needed to show any effect.

Long-term use of aspirin and NSAIDs and the risk of colorectal cancer
JAMA 2005; 294(8): 914–23

Several cohort and case control studies have consistently shown dose-related reductions of colorectal cancer in regular users of these drugs. Data from 80,000 people in the nurses' health study (running since 1976) found a reduction in colorectal cancer in those who regularly used aspirin, but the doses seem to be significantly higher than those needed to prevent cardiovascular disease.

Screening for bowel cancer

It is estimated that a 10-year screening programme would prevent 5,000 new cases and 3,000 deaths a year in the UK.

The Government made clear its commitment to screening for bowel cancer in the *NHS Plan* (2000), and the Colorectal Screening Pilot study began looking at faecal occult bloods (FOBs) and flexible sigmoidoscopies as options, building on original studies from Nottingham and Denmark. FOB screening could potentially reduce mortality from bowel cancer by 15%.

In October 2004 the Health Secretary announced that a national screening programme for bowel cancer will be rolled out to both men and women over 60 years of age from April 2006. This will be a phased plan and will be underpinned by £37.5 million of funding.

Home-testing kits will be sent every 2 years to men and women registered with a GP. They will have to collect a sample from three separate bowel movements within a 2-week period and then send the kit back (by post) to the laboratory. If the results are positive, patients will be offered a colonoscopy (this will be a separate route to the 2-week cancer referrals) through a local screening centre.

UK colorectal cancer screening pilot group. Results of the first round of a demonstration pilot of screening for colorectal cancer in the UK
BMJ 2004; 329: 133–5

Faecal occult blood screening (Cochrane Review 1998)

- Low sensitivity and specificity (tumour needs to be bleeding) in the range of 50–60%.

- Most extensively studied screening test for colorectal cancer.

- False-positives with red meat and vegetables rich in peroxidase.

- Several large randomised controlled trials have shown that FOB screening is feasible.

Flexible sigmoidoscopy

- Can detect 80% of colorectal cancers.

- Only detects cancers up to the splenic flexure (50% of cancers are proximal).

Tumour DNA

Gene expression profiles and molecular markers to predict recurrence of Duke's B colon cancer
J Clin Oncol 2004; 22(9): 1564–71

Genetic analysis of colorectal cancers is continuing behind the scenes, as tumour DNA can be detected from an early stage and may aid treatment decisions, especially around the use of adjuvant chemotherapy (currently only one-third of patients derive any benefit from this).

Coeliac disease

Banbury Coeliac Study
BMJ 1999; 318: 164–7

This study was set up to determine the under-diagnosis of coeliac disease. In the study 1,000 patients were tested for endomysial antibody (other antibody tests could include gliadin and reticulin). In total, 30 of these were positive with a positive biopsy result; 15 out of 30 patients presented with anaemia, and 25 out of 30 patients presented with non-gastrointestinal symptoms. It found that only around 20% of patients with coeliac disease are currently being diagnosed.

Prevalence of celiac disease in dyspeptic patients
Arq Gastroenterol 2005; 42(3): 153–6

This study looked at 142 patients being investigated for dyspepsia. A total of 30 patients were found to have patterns suggestive of coeliac disease, a prevalence of 1.4% in this study group (patients with irritable bowel syndrome are also know to have a higher prevalence). It suggests considering serological assays in this group of patients.

GPs can prescribe gluten-free foods to patients with coeliac disease or dermatitis herpetiformis, but must endorse the prescription 'ACBS' (According to Borderline Substance Act), otherwise the script may be queried. Compliance with a gluten-free diet has been shown to improve with medical follow-up. The British Society of Gastroenterology suggest this is done yearly.

Long-term complications of coeliac disease include small bowel lymphoma and osteoporosis (up to 50%). The Primary Care Society for Gastroenterology guidelines suggest a DEXA scan at the time of diagnosis and a repeat after the menopause for women, or at the age of 55 years for men. If a fragility fracture occurs at any age, then a scan should be performed.

The Coeliac Society produces an annual food list of gluten-free products, which is available to members (www.coeliac.co.uk).

The Department of Health advises prophylactic immunisation against *Pneumococcus* in coeliac disease patients over 2 years of age due to the risk of hyposplenism.

Mental health

The New Mental Health Act (revised from 1983)

The definition of a mental disorder is 'any disability or disorder of the mind or brain, whether permanent or temporary, which results in an impairment or disturbance of mental functioning'. Not only is the definition broad, but it is an emotive subject where patients and public have preconceived ideas, especially with regard to loss of rights. The reformed act goes some way towards addressing difficult issues, but it is important to remember that there is a distinct difference between treating mental disorders and exercising social control.

The White Paper *Reforming the Mental Health Act* (January 2001) is not yet law, although the draft Mental Health Bill was presented to Parliament in 2004. Certain elements have to be tested. The changes will ensure that the bill is compatible with human rights legislation.

A New Mental Health (and Public Protection) Act was first published in 1959, the main issues being that decisions on involuntary treatment for mental disorders became primarily a matter for doctors. In 1983, limits to medical discretion were set out.

The key issues with regard to mental health are listed below.

Risk of patients to themselves and others

- Care and treatment provided should reflect the best interest of the patient.

- Half the paper is devoted to high-risk patients.

- Perceived failures in community care are the main driving force.

Simpler template for formal assessment

- Assessment will be conducted by two doctors and an approved social worker (no change).

- The template will be set out in a formal care plan which must be of 'direct therapeutic benefit' or address the management of 'behaviours arising from the disorder'.
- After 28 days it will have to be reauthorised by the Mental Health Tribunal (a new independent body).
- It will be followed by a care and treatment order applicable in both civil and criminal justice which will be made by the Mental Health Tribunal or by a court.

Care and treatment in the community

- Care and treatment orders may apply to patients outside hospital.
- There will be contingency plans if patients refuse to take their medication in the community, to prevent patients becoming a risk to themselves and others.

Safeguards

- There is entitlement to free legal service.
- There is a statutory obligation for care plans.
- The Mental Health Tribunal is an independent body taking advice from the clinical team, patients, independent experts and other agencies. It is also concerned with long-term use of compulsory powers. It may exceptionally reserve the right not to accept the clinical supervisor's decision to discharge a patient if there is serious risk of harm to others.
- The New Commission for Mental Health has responsibilities for maintaining formal powers and looking after people subject to care and treatment orders.

Mental health legislation should respect decision-making capacity
BMJ 2005; 331: 1467–71 (Education and Debate)

This is a difficult article to summarise. It is worth reading to help understanding of this topic and is followed by two further commentaries. It discusses the issues around the ethics of mental health legislation, the ethics of autonomy and some of the difficulties with a person who has a mental capacity that is so seriously impaired that respect for their autonomy is no longer as important as their protection. The deprivation of a person's liberty is one of the most serious actions a state can take, this article will help you to understand the magnitude of such action when a person has committed no crime.

Implications of the law for GPs in England include the following.

- Increased workload for GPs with compulsory treatment orders.
- GPs may need to become involved in mental health tribunals, particularly for patients treated in the community.
- GP practices may be designated as places where compulsory treatment is administered.

Changing Minds: Every Family in the Land

This is a 5-year campaign organised by the Royal College of Psychiatrists to combat the stigmatisation of people with anxiety disorders, severe depression, dementia, schizophrenia, eating disorders, drug and alcohol dependencies.

Mental Illness: stigmatisation and discrimination within the medical profession is a report targeted at professionals as part of the campaign.

In 2001, the World Health Organization (WHO) published the first global profile of mental health services, which concluded that in most countries mental health is not taken seriously.

Admission under compulsion

This is only to be used where the patient is suffering from a mental disorder and cannot be persuaded to enter hospital voluntarily. Never use it lightly, and always keep comprehensive notes. Acceptance by the receiving hospital is necessary.

Section 2 (assessment)

- Should be used where possible (Section 4 may be more appropriate in general practice).
- The maximum length of stay is 28 days.
- It is applied for by an approved social worker or nearest relative.
- It is supported by two doctors (one of whom must be Section 12 approved and one of whom has knowledge of the patient). The two doctors need to examine the patient within 5 days of each other.

Section 3 (admission and treatment)

- Application is based on two medical recommendations.
- Length of stay is for 6 months initially, typically following on from a Section 2.

Section 4 (emergency in the community)

- The maximum length of admission is 72 hours.
- It is applied for by an approved social worker or nearest relative.
- It is supported by one doctor, who should have previous knowledge of the patient if possible. Both individuals must have seen the patient within 24 hours of admission.

National Service Framework for Mental Health (September 1999)

- At any one time one in six adults suffers from a mental illness (mainly anxiety or depression).

- One in 250 people have a psychotic illness, e.g. schizophrenia or bipolar affective disorder.

- Nine in 100 people who consult their GP with a psychiatric problem will be referred to specialist services.

- Mental health is one of four target areas in *Saving Lives: our healthier nation* and there is a specific target to reduce suicide by 20% by 2010.

- The NSF fleshes out policies in the White Paper *Modernising Mental Health Services*.

- An investment in mental health services of £700 million is planned over the next 3 years.

The NSF has five main areas and seven standards.

Mental health promotion (Standard 1)

1 Health and social services should:
   - promote mental health for all
   - combat discrimination against individual groups.

Primary care and access to services (Standards 2 and 3)

2 Any service user who contacts their primary healthcare team with a common mental health problem should:
   - have their mental health needs identified and assessed
   - be offered effective treatments and referral if required.

3 Any individual with a common mental health problem should:
   - be able to have 24-hour contact with social services
   - be able to use NHS Direct for first-level advice.

Effective services for people with severe mental illness (standards 4 and 5)

4 All mental health service users on care programmes should:
   - receive care that prevents or anticipates crisis and reduces risk
   - have written care plans that include action to be taken in a crisis, as well as GP advice if the patient needs additional help. These should be regularly reviewed by the co-ordinator
   - be able to access services 24 hours a day 365 days a year.

5 Each service user who is assessed as requiring a period of care away from their home should:
   - have access to an appropriate bed
   - be placed as close to home as possible
   - receive a copy of a written after-care plan on discharge.

Caring about carers (standard 6)

6 All individuals who provide regular and substantial care for a person on a care programme approach should:
- have an assessment of physical and mental needs annually
- have their own written care plan.

Preventing suicide (standard 7)

7 All standards 1 to 6, and in addition:
- supporting local prison staff in preventing suicide among prisoners
- ensuring the competence of staff
- developing local systems for suicide audit.

The overall performance will be assessed at national and local level in a number of ways:

- long-term improvement in psychological health of the population, as measured by the National Psychiatric Morbidity Survey

- reduction in suicide rates

- prescribing data

- access to psychiatric services and therapies

- experience of users

- reduction in the number of emergency admissions.

General opinions on the NSF

The physical health of people with severe mental illness
BMJ 2001; 322: 443–4

- It's about time!

- It is workable and clearly set out.

- On the whole there is an evidence base (but how can you audit discrimination?).

- Investment is planned, but it is never enough.

- It will need huge drive on staff recruitment, training and support.

- Patients and carers referred to as 'service users' − interesting!

- It ultimately relies on 24-hour access through NHS Direct, but is this really the best point of access for this sort of patient?

- Physical health needs are only highlighted with reference to the carers. We know that patients with severe mental illness have high rates of physical illness, which is often undetected, with twice the mortality of the general population.

BMJ 2002; 324: 61–2 (Editorial)

- It only covers adults up to 65 years of age (cf. discrimination issues). Elderly and young people/children will be addressed in separate service development programmes.
- It supports regional mental health development.
- Plans have been developed by region.
- Implementation team support.
- Bipolar affective disorder has been left out in the cold.
- Facilitators are in place to:
  - form a relationship with the primary healthcare team
  - encourage assessment of current practice
  - offer resources to assist process of change (e.g. guidelines)
  - promote teamwork and improve links
  - organise educational activity.

Br J Gen Pract 2000; 50: 626

Although facilitators have been shown to improve GP management in cerebrovascular accidents, heart disease and asthma, a randomised controlled trial of six practices with facilitators and six controls has shown that although recognition of mental illness was improved, there was no change in treatment or outcome. Debate at your leisure!

Dying for a drink
BMJ 2001; 323: 817–18

In this national confidential enquiry, 40% of people who committed suicide in England and Wales (who had been in contact with the NHS within 1 year of their death) had a history of alcohol misuse, and 19% also misused drugs.

This is a fundamental area to be targeted if we are to achieve the aims of section 7.

Suicide Prevention Strategy for England

www.doh.gov.org.uk/mentalhealth/exe-sum-intro.htm
www.nimhe.org.uk

- Around 5,000 people take their own life each year.
- Suicide is the most common cause of death in men under 35 years of age.
- Risk factors include the following:
  - male
  - living alone
  - unemployed
  - alcohol and drug misuse
  - mental illness.

The strategy was written to support the target set by the White Paper *Saving Lives: our healthier nation* and the NSF for Mental Health. The aim is to reduce death from suicide by at least 20% by 2010.

The goals of the programme are as follows:

- to reduce the risk to key high-risk groups
- to promote mental wellbeing in the wider population
- to reduce availability and lethality of suicide methods
- to improve reporting of suicide behaviour in the media
- to promote research on suicide prevention
- to improve monitoring of progress.

Anyone who self-harms requiring admission should have a follow-up visit by community mental health teams within 1 week. They should not be issued with repeat medication lasting more than 2 weeks.

Implementation will fall to the National Institute for Mental Health in England.

A qualitative study of health-seeking and primary care consultations prior to suicide
Br J Gen Pract 2005; Jul: 503–9

Half, or more, of people who take their own life do not consult a doctor in the month before their death. Family members and immediate social networks may play a key role in determining whether or not suicidal individuals seek help.

RCT of acute mental health care by a crisis resolution team: the north Islington crisis study
BMJ 2005; 331: 599–602

This study found that mental health crisis resolution teams can reduce hospital admissions.

Depression

- One in 20 people have clinical depression.
- Around 50% of depression is not diagnosed.

Br J Gen Pract 2000; 50: 284

Depression can be a disabling condition, and it is important to be aware of the symptoms and how the many faces of depression can touch every aspect of a person's life. GPs' diagnoses of depression have good levels of concordance with DSM-IV. However, we do still miss up to 50% of cases. This can be improved with a change in consultation style: asking open questions, making eye contact, not interrupting, etc.

DSM-IV diagnostic scale

Five of the following options should be present over a 2-week period for the diagnosis of major depression.

Depressed mood or irritability
Loss of interest or pleasure $\Big\}$ at least one of these symptoms

Appetite or weight loss
Sleep loss/change in sleep pattern
Psychomotor agitation or retardation
Fatigue/loss of energy $\Bigg\}$ three or four of these symptoms to make a total of five
Worthlessness or guilt
Poor concentration
Recurrent suicidal thoughts/thoughts of death

The above criteria are useful in differentiating between low mood and clinical depression. In chronic depressive illness (dysthymia), be aware that patients may not meet DSM-IV criteria but could still benefit from drug treatment in the short term.

Depression: management of depression in primary and secondary care NICE December 2004

This uses the International Classification of Diseases – version 10 (ICD-10). The recommendations are presented in the form of practical, stepped care (steps 1 to 5), starting with recognition of depression and going through treatment options based on severity of symptoms. The key priorities for implementation build on the NSF for Mental Health.

This is a very useful guide to read alongside the NICE Anxiety 2004 publication.

NICE guidelines for the management of depression *BMJ* 2005; 330: 267–8

This editorial outlines the views that the guidelines are clear for moderate to severe depression, but less so for mild to moderate depression (partly because of lack of understanding about what happens when individuals seek help for emotional problems).

Screening questionnaires

These are useful to aid diagnosis and monitor progress.

- *General Health Questionnaire*: designed for adults, it assesses inability to function normally.
- *Geriatric Depression Scale* (see below): designed for elderly people, it avoids somatic items.

- *Beck Depression Inventory*: designed for patients with more severe depression, it tackles suicidal thinking.

- *Edinburgh Postnatal Depression Scale*: more sensitive than other scales in postnatal women.

- *Abbreviated Mental Test Score* (see below): can be used as a guide to dementia.

- *Hamilton Depression Rating Scale*: not ideal for older people as it includes a number of somatic items that may be positive in older people who are not depressed.

Screening for depression in primary care
Br J Gen Pract 2005; Sept: 659–60

This is a sensible editorial exploring the practicalities of screening in primary care for an illness that may have no preclinical phase. The MaGPIe research group found that screening all attenders was far less effective than targeting patients at high risk.

Effect of the addition of a 'help' question in two screening questions on specificity for diagnosis of depression in general practice
BMJ 2005; 331: 884–6

The following three questions were asked of 1,025 consecutive patients receiving no psychotropic drugs and in whom substance misuse had been excluded.

- During the past month, have you often been bothered by feeling down, depressed or hopeless?

- During the past month have you often been bothered by little interest or pleasure in doing things?

- Is this something with which you would like help?

They had a sensitivity of 94% and specificity of 79%. The third question regarding help is what improved the specificity from 57% to 79%.

There has been much debate and work into improving the diagnosis of depression in general practice. The Hampshire Depression Project (*Lancet* 2000; 355: 185–91) looked at the effect of clinical practice guidelines and practice-based education on the detection and outcome of depression in primary care. They found that there was no improvement in detection when compared with usual care with no extra education/ protocols. Needless to say, GPs were criticised for not following guidelines.

The Defeat Depression Campaign was run by the Royal College of Psychiatrists and the Royal College of General Practitioners from 1992 to 1996 and was aimed at educating GPs in the recognition and management of depression, as well as enhancing public awareness.

New research by the Mental Health Foundation showed that GPs would like greater access to alternative treatments to medication, but lack of service provision or long waiting lists preclude this. They have produced two excellent leaflets on depression (including the role of exercise), which can be ordered online at www. mentalhealth.org.uk.

Abbreviated Mental Test Score (AMTS)

1	Age	0/1
2	Time (to nearest hour)	0/1
3	Address for recall at end – 42 West St	0/1
4	Year	0/1
5	Name of place (where test conducted)	0/1
6	Recognition of two people	0/1
7	Date of birth	0/1
8	Year of World War Two	0/1
9	Name of present monarch	0/1
10	Count backwards from 20 to 1	0/1

A score of <8 suggests impairment.

Geriatric Depression Scale

1	Are you basically satisfied with your life	Yes/**No**
2	Have you dropped many of your activities or interests	**Yes**/No
3	Do you feel that your life is empty	**Yes**/No
4	Do you often get bored	**Yes**/No
5	Are you in good spirits most of the time	Yes/**No**
6	Are you afraid that something bad is going to happen to you	**Yes**/No
7	Do you feel happy most of the time	Yes/**No**
8	Do you feel helpless	**Yes**/No
9	Do you prefer to stay at home rather than going out and doing new things	**Yes**/No
10	Do you feel you have more problems with memory than most	**Yes**/No
11	Do you think it is wonderful to be alive now	Yes/**No**
12	Do you feel pretty worthless the way you are now	**Yes**/No
13	Do you feel full of energy	Yes/**No**
14	Do you feel your situation is hopeless	**Yes**/No
15	Do you think that most people are better off than you are	**Yes**/No

Scoring: answers indicating depression are in bold type. Each scores 1 point. This scoring guidance should not be seen by the patient. A score ≥ 5 indicates probable depression.

Drug treatment in depression

You need to ask yourself what you are trying to achieve:

- improvement in mood, social and occupational function, quality of life

- reduction in morbidity and mortality

- prevention of a recurrence

- minimisation of adverse effects of treatment.

Antidepressants

Systematic reviews have shown that there is no clinically significant difference in effectiveness between different classes of drugs. All of them produce an improvement of 50–60%. On average, people on selective serotonin reuptake inhibitors (SSRIs) are less likely to stop treatment because of side effects. Because of this, SSRIs are now prescribed as first-line treatment (NICE, 2004). It is important to be aware of potential drug interactions, and to use recognised side effects to benefit the patient, e.g. if the patient is suffering from insomnia use those drugs with sedative side effects.

If there are no side effects the drug should be used for 6 weeks before changing class or increasing the dose. When stopping the drug, tail it off over 4 weeks (depending on the patient and their symptoms).

SSRIs and GI bleeding
BMJ 2005; 331: 529–30

This editorial explains the pathophysiological basis behind why SSRIs can cause gastrointestinal bleeding and why some patients would benefit from gastroprotection.

St John's Wort (Hypericum perforatum)

This is a low-grade monoamine oxidase inhibitor which is widely dispensed over the counter for low mood and depression. A systematic review of 27 studies (Cochrane Library 1999) concluded that it was more effective than placebo. However, various different preparations of *Hypericum* were used in each study.

Acute treatment of moderate to severe depression with St John's Wort: randomised controlled trial versus paroxetine
BMJ 2005; 330: 503–6

This study found that 90 mg/day of *Hypericum* extract (WS5570) three times a day (increased if there was no response after 6 weeks) was at least as effective after 42 days (assessed using the Hamilton Depression Scale) as paroxetine 20 mg (or 40 mg if the dose had to be increased).

Comparison of St John's Wort and imipramine for treating depression: randomised controlled trial
BMJ 2000; 321: 536–9

This study showed that *Hypericum* was therapeutically equivalent to imipramine but had a better side-effect profile. A total of 157 patients were scored on the Hamilton Depression Scale.

It is worth noting that *Hypericum* can induce liver enzymes and may interact with digoxin, theophylline, warfarin and the combined oral contraceptive pill (consult the *British National Formulary*). Also, different *Hypericum* products vary widely in composition.

Non-drug treatments (*Evidence-based Medicine* 2000)

Cognitive behavioural therapy (CBT)

This is a structured treatment aimed at changing dysfunctional beliefs and negative automatic thoughts that contribute to characterise depressive disorders. This form of treatment requires the therapist to have a high level of training.

The simple understanding is that CBT and problem solving are successful, whereas counselling is less so, although it does result in a high level of patient satisfaction. More recent studies looking at long-term outcome have on the whole found no difference between groups.

Cognitive therapy for prevention of suicidal attempts: randomised controlled trial
JAMA 2005; 294(5): 263–4

This was a randomised controlled trial (either 10 sessions of CBT or enhanced usual service) of 120 patients who had recently attempted to commit suicide. CBT was found to be effective at preventing further suicide attempts.

The future

Urinary screening may allow neurochemical profiling of depression subtypes, enabling more rational prescribing of antidepressants.

Schizophrenia

The first description of schizophrenia appeared in the eighteenth century. It has a 1% lifetime prevalence, with 25% of patients being cared for by their GP. The diagnosis is made on the basis of the WHO International Classification of Disease (ICD-10), which looks for clear evidence of past or present psychosis, absence of prominent affective symptoms and a minimum duration of illness. We also need to look for negative symptoms such as blunted affect or poor motivation.

Schneider's first-rank symptoms are summarised below:

- auditory hallucinations
- thought withdrawal or insertion
- thought broadcasting
- somatic passivity
- feelings or actions that are perceived as being under external control
- delusional perceptions.

How to manage first episode of schizophrenia
BMJ 2000; 321: 522

- The early stages of the disease form can predict the course and outcome of the illness.

- Early treatment may result in better prognosis and functional outcome. This is not as easy as it sounds, given the insidious nature of the condition as well as the reluctance to make such an early diagnosis.

- Around 70% of people will relapse within 5 years after the first attack. Therefore early withdrawal of treatment is not recommended.

- Effective treatment consists of the following:
  - a multidisciplinary team
  - drugs to control symptoms (no specific recommendations)
  - 'intensive' community rehabilitation ⎫
  - family therapy   ⎬ improve long-term social functioning after acute phase
  - psychological work, e.g. CBT.   ⎭

A randomised multicentre trial of integrated versus standard treatment for patients with a first episode of psychotic illness
BMJ 2005; 331: 586–7

This randomised trial of 547 patients in Copenhagen found that patients who received integrated treatment (2 years of assertive community treatment with family involvement and social skills training) had significantly less substance misuse, better adherence to and more satisfaction with treatment.

The new atypicals/antipsychotics

Schizophr Res 1999; 35: 51–68

There is substantial evidence that these drugs achieve good results with the positive symptoms. Even so, up to 30% of patients do not respond to psychopharmacology and negative symptoms are even less responsive. There is some evidence that the new antipsychotics reduce the rate of relapse during maintenance treatment.

The side-effect profile seems to be better, with fewer extra-pyramidal side effects. Note that clozapine decreases the white cell count and the latter therefore needs to be monitored.

The new antipsychotics should be considered as first-line treatment in newly diagnosed cases, where there has been no response to first-line therapy or where extra-pyramidal side effects have been a problem.

Non-compliance is a complex issue, but the new dissolve-in-the-mouth tablet goes some way to addressing this.

These drugs are insoluble in oil so are unlikely to be available as a depot formulation.

Prevention of schizophrenia

Yale University is recruiting people with a strong family history of schizophrenia or who show early signs of psychotic behaviour in order to look at the effects of olanzapine. Oxford University attempted a similar study some years ago but had difficulty in recruiting and allocating groups because of lack of understanding of the predictive power of clinical signs.

Summary of NICE schizophrenia guidelines, December 2002

The guidelines are relevant to adults over 18 years of age and to those diagnosed with schizophrenia below the age of 60 years. There are three phases.

1 Initiation of treatment (first episode):
   - early referral to secondary care and involvement of other services
   - early treatment – suggests discussion with psychiatrist and urgent referral. Consider atypicals (e.g. olanzapine) as first-line treatment.

2 Treatment of acute episode:
   - single drug – administer at *BNF* dose range for a minimum of 6 weeks and monitor the response
   - may need rapid tranquillisation
   - be aware of side effects, e.g. risk of diabetes and weight gain with some atypicals
   - address other needs – psychological, social, occupational, etc.
   - there is a high risk of relapse – if treating a relapse you need to continue treatment for 1–2 years and slowly withdraw treatment thereafter, monitoring for 2 years after the last acute episode.

3 Promoting recovery (primary care):
   - care register (essential)
   - monitor mental health and treatment alongside secondary care
   - consider referral in the following circumstances:
     - problem with compliance
     - poor response to treatment
     - suspected co-morbid substance misuse
     - increased risk to self or others
     - new to practice list – for assessment and care programme
     - service user prefers not to receive care from GP.

Document everything clearly.

The following are essential across all phases:

- optimism

- get help early

- assessment

- working in partnership

- consent

- accurate information

- addressing language and culture

- addressing the issue of advance directives (although limited in schizophrenia).

Eating disorders

The life time prevalence of eating disorders in young women is as follows (note that there is an even social class distribution):

- anorexia nervosa: 0.5–3.7%

- bulimia nervosa: 1.1–4.2%.

Up to 20% will die as a result of their illness.
   Many people do not ask for help, so as GPs we can play a vital role in the detection of these disorders. Recognised risk factors include genetic factors (we don't know what is inherited, possibly a vulnerable personality type), cultural values, childhood obesity, early onset of puberty, adverse life experiences, extreme shyness, bullying, family functional style and low self-esteem.

American Psychiatric Association 1994

In diagnosis, if the diagnostic criteria for both bulimia and anorexia are met, the diagnosis of anorexia takes precedence.
   Early diagnosis and intervention give better outcome. Cognitive behavioural therapy and SSRIs have both been shown to improve short-term outcome compared with placebo, but it is not yet clear if remission rates are reduced (**Cochrane Library**).
   Standards 2 and 3 of the National Service Framework for Mental Health outline the need to improve healthcare for patients with anorexia nervosa and bulimia nervosa.

The SCOFF questionnaire: assessment of a new screening tool for eating disorders
BMJ 1999; 319: 1467–8

This was designed at St George's Hospital, London, by Dr J Morgan and colleagues in order to give specialists a simple screening tool with which to identify eating disorders. It consists of five questions, and 1 point is scored for each 'Yes' answer. A score of >2 indicates a likely problem.

- Do you make yourself **S**ick because you feel uncomfortably full?

- Do you worry you have lost **C**ontrol over how much you eat?

- Have you recently lost more than **O**ne stone in a 3-month period?

- Do you believe yourself to be **F**at when others say you are too thin?

- Would you say that **F**ood dominates your life?

The researchers compared this tool with more lengthy questionnaires and obtained excellent results of 100% sensitivity and 87.5% specificity (12.5% false-positive rate).

The SCOFF questionnaire and clinical interview for eating disorders in general practice: comparative study
BMJ 2002; 325: 755–6

This study looked at the use of the SCOFF questionnaire in identifying patients in primary care. It found that the questionnaire detected all women with diagnosed anorexia and bulimia. In summary, it concluded that it was an efficient tool for detecting eating disorders in adults.

Counselling in general practice

Around 51% of general practices have an on-site counsellor.

Counselling is designed to help people work on their problems and become more skilled in helping themselves. It is a disciplined psychological intervention requiring specialist training in the different styles (e.g. directive, informative, confrontational, supportive, etc.). There is documented evidence that, if selected appropriately, it is effective. Counsellors have their own professional code of ethics and practice, and they must hold a current membership of a professional body, e.g. the British Association for Counselling and Psychotherapy.

Appropriate referral and assessment are essential for cost-effective intervention. Most counselling consists of 6 to 12 sessions.

Suitable candidates for brief focal counselling include those who:

- are able to express feelings and thoughts

- are able to trust the counsellor

- have mild to moderate difficulties, e.g. depression, relationship problems, anxiety, bereavement, emotional or psychological difficulties

- are able to bear disturbing or conflicting feelings.

Unsuitable candidates include those who:

- have moderate to severe difficulties, e.g. schizophrenia, dementia, substance abuse, personality disorders, risk of suicide

- are silent or withdrawn

- are prone to over intellectualisation

- have no close relationships

- lack the ability to think about self.

Counselling in general practice
Drug Ther Bull 2000; 38(7): 49–52

There is currently marked regional variation in the UK, which may change with primary care groups/trusts and National Service Frameworks. There are relatively few randomised controlled trials comparing counselling with usual GP care. However, a meta-analysis of four randomised controlled trials suggests 'statistically better' psychological symptom level after treatment than if just receiving GP care.

Chronic fatigue syndrome

For a review of chronic fatigue syndrome, see *BMJ* **2000; 320: 292–6**.

Chronic fatigue syndrome (CFS), also known as myalgic encephalitis (ME), is defined as disabling fatigue associated with other symptoms, e.g. musculoskeletal pain, sleep disturbance, impaired concentration and headaches. The cause is not understood.

The prevalence is currently 0.2–2.6%, and only one-third of patients with CFS meet the criteria of the Centre for Disease Control for CFS.

Treatment with antidepressants may be useful, especially if the condition is associated with depression, insomnia or myalgia.

A 37 kDa 2–5A binding protein as a potential biochemical marker for chronic fatigue syndrome
Am J Med 2000; 108: 99–105

This study found that a polypeptide involved in the antiviral response was more common in CFS. This may be of help in the future when trying to distinguish the syndrome from depression and other diseases.

A further study (*Neurology* **2005; 5: 23**) has confirmed similar findings. The five proteins isolated are alpha-1-macroglobulin, amyloid precursor-like protein 1, keratin 16, orosomucoid 2 and pigment epithelium-derived factor.

Treatment of CFS

Exercise

There have been several trials looking at graded exercise programmes over the past ten years.

A randomised controlled graded exercise trial for CFS: outcomes and mechanisms of change
J Health Psychol 2005; 10(2): 245–59

In this study, 49 patients were randomised to either a 12-week exercise programme or standard medical care. Graded exercise appears to be effective, operating in part by reducing the degree to which patients focus on their symptoms.

Cognitive behavioural therapy

A systematic review of three randomised controlled trials found that if CBT is delivered by highly skilled therapists in specialist centres there is a good outcome (Cochrane Library 1998) over a period of 6–12 months.

Treatment for CFS
Occ Med (London) **2005; 55(1): 32–9**

This was a limited meta-analysis, but found that the most promising outcomes were seen with CBT and graded exercise therapy. Pharmacological therapies were found to be less effective.

Medically unexplained symptoms

Drug Ther Bull **2001; 39(1): 5**
Around one in five new consultations are by patients with physical symptoms for which there is no organic cause. In a third of cases the symptoms persist and can cause distress and disability.

General practice is about dealing with symptoms that don't fit the disease model. Do not make the mistake of labelling symptoms MUS (medically unexplained symptoms) until a thorough clinical assessment and appropriate investigations have been carried out.

It is thought that, although by definition the cause is unknown, these symptoms are due to a complex interaction of biological, psychological, social and cultural factors.

Understanding the narratives of people who live with medically unexplained illness
Patient Educ Couns **2005; 56(2): 205–10**

This paper identified three features of patients' narratives: a chaotic history of the illness narrative; concerns that their symptoms were all in their mind; and their status as medical orphans. There was genuine concern to secure some form of ongoing medical and social support.

Management

It is important to acknowledge the symptoms and distress, and to provide continuity of care.

Management of medically unexplained symptoms (Editorial)
BMJ **2005; 330: 4–5**

This is a discussion of some of the issues and options available. It highlights some of the essential elements in medical models: to make the patient feel understood, then to broaden the agenda and finally to negotiate a new understanding of the symptoms including psychosocial factors.

Antidepressants

These can be useful, especially if the patient is experiencing pain or difficulty in sleeping, whether or not they are depressed. Benefit is usually seen in 1–7 days (i.e. quickly!). The number needed to treat is 3.

Reattribution

This involves demonstrating understanding of the patient's complaints by taking a history of related physical, mood and social factors. Making the patient feel understood and making the link between symptoms and psychological problems.

Cognitive behavioural therapy

This has been shown in systematic review to be beneficial, particularly in reducing physical symptoms.

Beyond somatisation: a review of the understanding and treatment of medically unexplained physical symptoms
Br J Gen Pract **2003; 53: 233–41**

This review article looks at the evidence for complex interactions of physical and cognitive processes. It discusses the complex adaptive system, a model that looks at internal and external interaction.

Frequent attenders

This is usually a different group of people to those with medically unexplained symptoms.

The average GP attendance per patient is three to four times per year.

Characteristics of high attenders include the following:

- multiple health problems
- lower social class
- medically unexplained symptoms
- belief that reattendance is necessary to get the right treatment.

Br J Gen Pract 2001; 51: 987–94

This study showed that psychosocial, lifestyle and health status variables help in predicting high attendance among adults.

Elderly care

National Service Framework for Older People

This was published in March 2001 (www.doh.gov.uk/nsf/olderpeople.htm). It is an action plan to improve health and social services for older people wherever they live. It focuses on the following:

- rooting out age discrimination
- patient-centred care

- promoting older people's health and independence/an active life

- management of specific clinical conditions, with timely access to specialist care.

The eight standards are listed below.

1 Root out age discrimination, providing care on the basis of clinical need alone.

2 Person-centred care – treat patients as individuals. There will be a single assessment process with integrated provision of services and GPs will mainly be involved in the contact assessment.

3 Intermediate care – to enable early hospital discharge and to prevent premature or unnecessary admission to long-term residential care.

4 General hospital care – delivered through appropriate specialist care, by staff with the skills to meet their needs.

5 Stroke – the NHS will take action to prevent strokes (primary and secondary), it will provide treatment by specialist stroke services with a multidisciplinary programme of secondary prevention and rehabilitation.

6 Falls – the NHS and councils will take action to prevent falls and reduce resultant fractures or other injuries. Advice will be provided through specialised falls services.

7 Mental health in older people – there will be access to integrated mental health services (for patients and carers).

8 Promotion of health and active life in older age.

As well as the eight standards listed above, there are five other major projects under way to improve quality, availability and consistency of services.

- Changes in long-term care funding, including availability of NHS nursing care.

- Expansion of intermediate care (and community equipment) services.

- Establishment of Care Direct to provide comprehensive information and ease of access to health, housing, social care and social security.

- Various initiatives (retirement health check, flu immunisations) to help older people stay healthy.

- Use of Section 31 Health Act 1999 to promote joint working between NHS and social services.

Progress will be overseen by the NHS Modernisation Board and the Older People's Taskforce.

The Department of Health will publish the *Information Strategy for Older People,* which is due out later this year (2006) and will describe how GPs will be supported in achieving this.

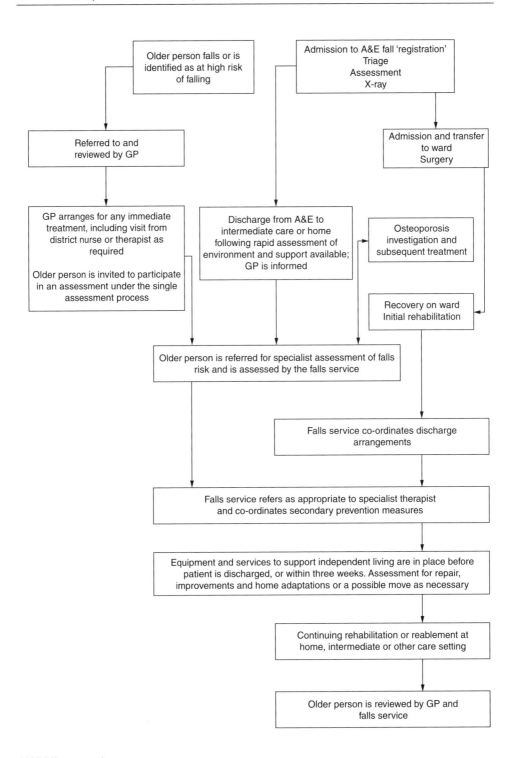

NSF falls care pathway.

Falls

- Falls are the leading cause of accidental death in people over 75 years of age; treatment of fractures alone costs the NHS £1.7 billion per year (DoH 2003).

- Every year 33–50% of people over 65 years of age suffer a fall (the percentage increases with age), of whom 20% will need medical help and 10% will have sustained a fracture.

- The current blood pressure targets seem to be causing an increase in falls due to postural hypotension and medication.

How can we help older people not fall again? Implementing the Older Person's NSF Falls Standard Six
Department of Health 2003

This is a comprehensive overview of reasoning and evidence behind current think-ing around falls prevention, as well as the evidence behind the case for funding a falls prevention strategy locally. NICE has produced guidelines to support the Government.

NICE 2004

One of the most important things to understand in this document is how you would offer a multifactoral assessment of falls by assessing:

- fall history; gait, balance, mobility and muscle weakness
- osteoporosis risk
- visual and cognitive impairment
- urinary incontinence
- home hazards
- cardiovascular examination and medication review.

Promoting health and function in an ageing population
BMJ 2001; 322: 728–9

This article reviews the evidence for strategies promoting health and function. It concludes that it is necessary to take into account social, mental, economic and environmental determinants of health in old age. Most health benefits can be gained from regular physical activity of moderate intensity, and substantial gains could be made by promoting health and fitness throughout life.

GPs should:

- review repeat prescriptions
- consider physiotherapy referral
- consider occupational therapy referral to reduce home hazards

- consider a joint meeting with the relevant primary healthcare team members for individual cases
- consider asking if there have been any falls in the past 12 months at routine reviews.

Simple measures could reduce falls by a half (Department of Health 2003):

- ensure that footwear fits correctly – no 'sloppy slippers'
- instal night lights to reduce night falls, e.g. pressure mats next to the bed to trigger the lighting
- practising Tai chi could help balance and strength.

Randomised controlled trial of prevention of falls in older people aged ≥75 with severe visual impairment: the VIP trial
BMJ 2005; 331: 817–20

This trial assessed the cost-effectiveness of a home safety programme and a home exercise programme to reduce falls and injuries in 391 older patients with impaired vision. The home safety programme reduced falls and was the most cost-effective, compared with the exercise programme, in this group of patients.

Patients with recurrent falls attending A&E benefit from multifactoral intervention – a randomised controlled trial
Age and Ageing 2005; 34(2): 162–8

A total of 313 cognitively intact patients attending A&E with fall-related injuries and who had had at least one other fall in the preceding 12 months were randomised to either normal A&E care or a post-fall medical, physiotherapy and occupational therapy. There were 36% fewer falls in the intervention group.

Residronate sodium therapy for prevention of hip fractures in men 65 years or older after stroke
Arch Intern Med 2005; 165(15): 1743–8

This was an 18-month randomised double-blind trial of 280 men post stroke. Residronate increased bone mineral density and reduced hip fractures due to falls in this group.

Dementia

Dementia is the chronic deterioration of intellect and personality.

- Around 5% of people over 65 years of age have some form of dementia.
- Around 20% of people over 80 years of age have some form of dementia.
- One in seven elderly people with dementia are in residential care.
- It is important to diagnose dementia early and to identify the type of dementia to improve care and reduce morbidity for our patients and their carers.

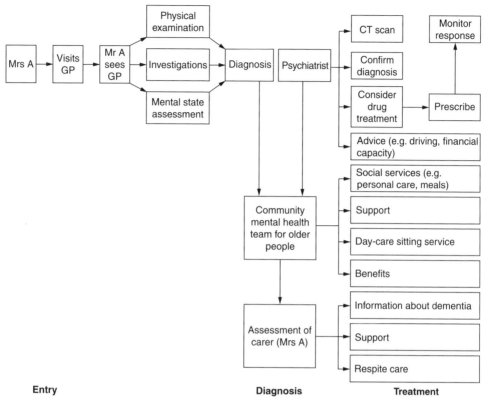

Entry   **Diagnosis**   **Treatment**
Mr A is an 84-year-old former school teacher who is living with his wife. She has arthritis and has
begun to worry about her husband's forgetfulness.
The single assessment process could initiate referral to the GP, or the diagnosis itself could
initiate an assessment.

NSF flow chart for dementia.

The Mental Health Foundation has published a report entitled *Tell Me the Truth,* which states that most people who develop dementia are not usually told what is wrong with them. It is this information that, although initially difficult to accept, helps patients to understand the changes in themselves and helps them to adapt.

NICE is in the consultation period of developing guidelines for dementia.

The limited utility of MMSE in screening older people >75 for dementia in primary care
Br J Gen Pract 2002; 52: 1002–3

The Mini Mental State Examination (MMSE) is recommended as a screening instrument for dementia. A total of 709 patients completed the MMSE, and it was found that it had an 86% false-positive rate for identifying dementia in primary care (202 were validated against GMS-AGECAT diagnostic system) when used with a weighting of 26/30. However, if a cut-off of 21 was used the false-positive rate dropped to 59%.

Are GPs able to accurately diagnose dementia and identify Alzheimer's disease? A comparison with an out patient memory clinic
Br J Gen Pract **2000; 50: 311–12**

This is a cross-sectional study from the Netherlands. GPs were able to assess the firmness of their own dementia diagnosis, i.e. appropriate selection for referral. They were less good at determining the type of dementia.

Alzheimer's disease

This is the most common form of dementia in the UK (accounting for around 60% of cases). There are about 340,000 cases in the UK. In rare cases it is inherited via the AD gene. There are also connections to the Apo-E gene, but no useful diagnostic or prognostic test is yet available.

Current management focuses on accurate diagnosis, providing appropriate services, supporting carers and treating non-cognitive problems.

Drugs for Alzheimer's disease

Three cholinesterase inhibitors have been licensed in the UK for mild to moderate Alzheimer's disease: donezipil, rivastigmine and galantamine. They have all been shown to improve cognitive function, global outcome and activities of daily living. More recent evidence is now starting to cast doubt on these original findings.

Cholinesterase inhibitors for patients with Alzheimer's disease: systematic review of randomised clinical trials
BMJ **2005; 331: 321–5**

The authors looked at randomised controlled trials of donepezil, rivastigmine and galantamine from 1989–2004 and found that the scientific basis for recommending these drugs was questionable.

Summary of NICE Guidelines (January 2001) for cholinesterase inhibitors (under review)

- Diagnosis must be made by a specialist (according to criteria).

- Activities of daily living, cognition, global and behavioural functioning must be assessed prior to treatment. The MMSE score must be >12.

- Treatment can be continued if there is an improvement/no deterioration in the MMSE 2–4 months after reaching maintenance dose.

- Patients should be reviewed every 6 months.

- Compliance must be ensured.

- GPs may take over prescribing under an agreed shared-care protocol.

It is thought that the revised guidelines will recommend withdrawal of anti-cholinesterase inhibitors and that Ebixa should be licensed for moderate to severe dementia.

It is also thought that drug costs may be offset by delaying the need for residential care. Specialist memory clinics/secondary care need to expand (these clinics are recommended in the National Service Framework for Older People).

Glutamatergic modulators are a new treatment on the market and are not yet included in the guidelines.

Other treatments

1 *Selegiline and vitamin E*: treatment with either was found to slow progression of the disease. The Cochrane Review 2000 found that selegiline was better than placebo in improving cognitive function, behavioural disturbance and mood.

2 *Vitamin C and vitamin E for Alzheimer's disease*: **Ann Pharmacother 2005; 39: 2073–9** concluded that vitamin C and E supplements do not have the supporting evidence to be recommended for use in Alzheimer's disease.

3 *Ginkgo biloba* (40 mg three times a day): one systematic review (of eight randomised trials) reported that *ginkgo biloba* improved cognitive function and was well tolerated in patients with Alzheimer's disease (**Clin Drug Invest 1999; 17: 301–8**).

4 *Reality orientation*: this involves presenting information designed to reorientate a person in time, place and person. It may be a notice board giving day, date and time or a member of staff reorientating the patient at each contact. **Clinical Evidence** found one systematic review of small randomised controlled trials that showed improvement in cognitive function and behaviour compared to no treatment.

Miscellaneous factors
Midlife vascular risk factors and Alzheimer's disease in later life: longitudinal population-based study
BMJ 2001; 322: 1447–57

This study found that raised systolic blood pressure and high cholesterol, especially in combination and in mid-life, increased the risk of Alzheimer's disease in later life. This could have future implications in patient management.

1 *Exercise*

Leisure-time physical activity at midlife and the risk of dementia and Alzheimer's disease
Lancet 2005; 4(11): 705–11

This was a study of 1,239 people aged 65–79 years, which found that exercising at least twice a week was associated with a 50% lower relative risk of dementia and 60% lower risk of Alzheimer's disease. This was especially so (once adjusted for other factors) in carriers of the APOE gene.

2 *Statins*

Statin use and the risk of incidental dementia: the cardiovascular health study
Arch Neurol 2005; 62: 1047–51

Although several other papers have found a possible reduction in the risk of developing dementia with statin use, this study of 2,800 patients found that the incidence of dementia among statin users was the same as for those not using statins.

3 *Hormone replacement therapy*: there is evidence that HRT may be beneficial. One study found that women who had been on HRT for 3 years were 40% less likely to develop Alzheimer's disease, and for those who had been on it for 10 years the reduction was 60% (*Lancet* 2002; 288: 2123–9). However, it is feasible that HRT may increase the risk of vascular dementia from associated strokes.

4 *Diet*

Fish, meat and the risk of dementia: cohort study
BMJ 2002; 325: 932–3

Data drawn from PAQUID (a French epidemiological survey) were used, and it was found that people who eat fish or seafood at least once a week were at lower risk of developing dementia, including Alzheimer's disease.

5 *Non-steroidal anti-inflammatory drugs*

NSAIDs and the risk of Alzheimer's disease
NEJM 2001; 345: 1515–21

There is a hypothesis that inflammatory mechanisms play a part in Alzheimer's disease. In this study, 6,989 residents in Rotterdam aged over 55 years with no evidence of dementia were included, with a follow-up of 8 years, and the MMSE and Geriatric Mental State Examination were administered. It found that as NSAID use (other than aspirin) increased, the relative risk of Alzheimer's disease fell from 0.95 to 0.2. The type of NSAID did not influence this effect. No benefit was found in vascular dementia.

More recent studies seem to support these results, although to date this is the largest study of its kind.

Detection
Detection of Alzheimer's disease and dementia in the pre-clinical phase: population-based cohort
BMJ 2003; 326: 245–7

This study looked at three steps: self-reported memory complaints, test of global cognitive function and specific cognitive tests. Although only 18% of people in the pre-clinical phase were identified, the test had a positive predictive value of 85–100% for these cases.

Parkinson's disease

The prevalence of Parkinson's disease is one in 1,000 at 55 years (the average age of onset) and one in 200 in those over 65 years of age.

On the whole, treatment is best resisted unless there is a functional disability. No drugs have been found to delay progression.

Clinical Practice. Diagnosis and initial management of Parkinson's disease
NEJM **2005; 353(10): 1021–7**

This is one of the most up-to-date reviews, although *Clinical Evidence* and many other sites will give you more information.

Guidelines for management of Parkinson's disease in primary care by the Primary Care Task Force are available from: Parkinson's disease, 215 Vauxhall Bridge Rd, London SW1 1EJ.

Surgery

Thalamotomy, pallidotomy, deep brain stimulation or foetal nigral implants are all being trialled. Initial results in selected groups have shown an improvement in contralateral symptoms of tremor and bradykinesis.

Depression

This is common in Parkinson's disease (up to 50% of cases). It is thought to have neurobiological manifestations rather than being a purely emotional response to the disease (*J Neurol Neurosurg Psychiatry* **1999; 67: 492–6**).

Dementia

It is recognised that patients with Parkinson's disease have an increased risk of developing dementia.

Prognosis of PD: risk of dementia and mortality: Rotterdam study
Arch Neurol **2005; 62(8): 1265–7**

This study found that the risk of dementia was more prevalent if patients carried the APOE episton allele. The dementia risk was also dependent on disease duration.

New advances

Gene therapy
Science **2002; 298: 425–9**

So far this has only been carried out on rats. The first human trial has just been approved in the USA.

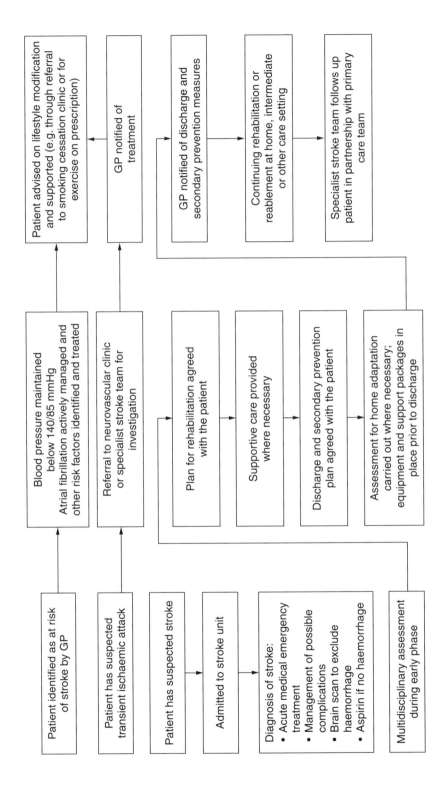

NSF stroke care pathway.

Dietary supplements
Arch Neurol 2002; 59: 1541–50

Co-enzyme Q10 may reduce functional decline in Parkinson's disease.

Stroke

Stroke is defined as a sudden loss of neurological function lasting for more than 24 hours. A transient ischaemic attack (TIA) lasts for less than 24 hours. Stroke is covered by Standard 5 of the National Standard Framework for Older People.

- The incidence of stroke is 2 in 1,000 (double this in those aged 45–84 years).

- It is the third most common cause of death in the UK and the greatest single cause of disability, affecting 130,000 people per year.

- Around 80% of all strokes are ischaemic.

- Around 50% of patients are physically dependent on others 6 months after the event.

- The incidence of TIA is 0.4 in 1,000 (the future risk of stroke is 10% in the first year and 5% thereafter). There is a 1–2% risk of a myocardial infarction following TIA.

A simple score (ABCD) to identify individuals at high early risk of stroke after TIA
Lancet 2005; 366: 29–36

Deciding which patients need emergency assessment following a TIA is an important part of our initial management in general practice (although the gold standard is that all should be investigated within 7 days), and this outlines a simple scoring system to assist decision making.
  The criteria used were:

ABCD	Meaning	Question	Score
A	Age	<60 years	0
		>60 years	1
B	Blood pressure	Systolic >140 mmHg and/or	1
		Diastolic >90 mmHg/l	
C	Clinical features	Unilateral weakness	2
		Speech disturbance, no weakness	1
		Other	0
D	Duration of symptoms	60 minutes	2
		10–59 minutes	1
		<10 minutes	0

A score >5/8 was predictive (in up to 24% of the 190 patients) of a subsequent stroke within 7 days of a TIA. As this is suggested for use as part of the initial assessment it does not factor in smoking history/pack years or cholesterol.

National Service Framework for Older People: Standard 5 – Stroke

Outcome for stroke patients is better and their stay in hospital is usually shorter if they are cared for by specialist teams in stroke units. It specifically states:

- people who are thought to have had a stroke should have access to diagnostic and specialist stroke services
- subsequently they, and their carers, should participate in a multidisciplinary programme of secondary prevention and rehabilitation (e.g. speech therapy, occupational therapy, physiotherapy, social services, district nurse support, etc.).

Prevention (primary and secondary)

Hypertension
Hypertension accounts for up to 50% of ischaemic strokes. The British Hypertension Society guidelines state that hypertension persisting for more than 1 month after a stroke should be treated. Stroke risk can be reduced by up to 40% if the diastolic blood pressure is reduced by 6 mmHg or the systolic BP is reduced by 10–12 mmHg (irrespective of whether the BP is elevated or not).

Role of blood pressure and other variables in the differential cardiovascular event rates noted in the Anglo-Scandinavian Cardiac Outcomes Trial – blood pressure-lowering arm (ASCOT-BPLA)
Lancet **2005; 366: 869–71**

This study showed significantly lower rates of stroke in the amlodipine vs. the atenolol regimen. The significance was not fully understood and may be statistical rather than a real finding in this group of patients.

Heart Outcomes prevention Study (HOPE)
NEJM **2002; 347: 145–53**

This study of ramipril showed a 32% decrease in stroke in patients with controlled blood pressure, highlighting that all patients should have an angiotensin converting enzyme inhibitor irrespective of their blood pressure.

Antiplatelet drugs
Prescribing antiplatelets in primary care was the topic of an *MeReC Bulletin* in July 2005 (www.npc.nhs.uk). It is summarised in the cardiovascular disease chapter of this book.

Antiplatelet agents in secondary prevention of stroke: a perspective
Stroke **2005; 36: 2034–6**

Aspirin is the treatment of choice for secondary prevention of stroke, especially if the first was a non-disabling stroke or TIA (around 24% reduction in subsequent events). No one dose is more effective than another (dispersible vs. enteric-coated affectivity is being debated; dispersible is cheaper than enteric-coated). This paper suggests taking another look at antiplatelet compounds rather than funding the ongoing 'drug war'.

Antiplatelet therapy for preventing stroke in patients with non-valvular atrial fibrillation and no previous history of stroke or TIA
Cochrane Database **2005; 19: 4: CD001925**

Aspirin appears to reduce stroke and major vascular events in patients with non-valvular atrial fibrillation (dose 75–325 mg). For primary prevention among atrial fibrillation patients, about 10 strokes per 1,000 patients would be prevented.

Anticoagulation in atrial fibrillation
Atrial fibrillation (AF) increases the risk of stroke sixfold. Warfarin was previously the drug of choice for prevention of stroke in AF. Several randomised controlled trials confirmed the benefit and low complication rate (0.4%). The number needed to treat to prevent one stroke was 11.

Systematic review of long-term anticoagulation of antiplatelet treatment in patients with non-rheumatic atrial fibrillation
BMJ **2001; 322: 321–6**

The review found no added benefit in *non-rheumatic AF*. Previous meta-analyses had not included these trials. There were 3,298 patients (thought to be too low a number, as around 5,000 are needed). Individual trials were small and used slightly different international normalised ratios to monitor warfarin. Around 45% of patients were more likely to bleed on warfarin (even within the controlled setting of the trial). It was concluded that there was no obvious benefit gained from using warfarin.

Cholesterol
If a patient has had a stroke but does not have coronary heart disease (CHD), the benefits of reduction of cholesterol are less clear. Statins are indicated as part of a secondary prevention treatment plan for patients following a stroke or TIA. However, guidance on statin use for primary prevention is to be widened by NICE to include patients with a 10-year CHD risk of 20% (it may be extended further to a 10-year cardiovascular risk of 20% – this would mean an extra 3 million adults would qualify for treatment).

The Heart Protection Study
Lancet **2002; 360: 7–20**

This study of the treatment of high-risk CHD patients with simvastatin found that simvastatin reduced the incidence of stroke by up to 25%.

The role of statins in the prevention of ischaemic stroke
Curr Atheroscler Rep **2005; 7(5): 364–8**

Stroke incidence in patients taking statins has reduced in patients being treated for ischaemic heart disease, diabetes and hypertension, and also (though to a lesser extent) in patients who have had a previous stroke (the article discusses the two most recent meta-analyses). Statins are thought to work by lowering LDL, stabilising plaques, improving endothelial function and nitric oxide bioavailability, and inhibiting inflammatory responses.

Carotid endarterectomy

If there is a symptomatic stenosis, the benefit of surgery relates to the degree of stenosis. This is classified as mild, moderate or severe (Cochrane Review, 2003). Carotid endarterectomy for asymptomatic carotid stenosis reduces the risk of stroke by 30% over 3 years (Cochrane Review, 2005).

See also www.eGuidelines.co.uk for information based on the Royal College of Physician's *National Clinical Guidelines for Stroke Management* (published in 2002). Its most recent publication is *Stroke Transfer of Care* (August 2005), which takes you through care and rehabilitation in primary care.

Diabetes

- The prevalence of diabetes in the UK is 3% (10% in those over 65 years of age).

- There are 33,000 deaths per year due to diabetes.

- Life expectancy is reduced by up to 20 years in type 1 and 10 years in type 2 diabetes.

- Coronary heart disease is increased fivefold and stroke is increased threefold.

Diabetes is a complex multisystem disease and for effective management you need, preferably, a co-ordinated patient-centred approach with set standards and a computerised register. It is a common disease, and it is estimated that its incidence will rise by 25% over the next decade due to the ageing population, obesity, sedentary lifestyle, etc. St Vincent's declaration, ratified by the WHO regional committee for Europe in 1991, set aspirations and goals for reducing the impact of diabetes.

Recent changes relating to diabetes include the following:

- new WHO classifications (June 2000)

- NICE guidelines

- the British Diabetic Association has been renamed Diabetes UK

- the National Service Framework for Diabetes (2003).

Diagnosis

The criteria for diagnosis were agreed by the World Health Organization in June 2000.

1 Diabetic symptoms with random venous glucose concentration >11.1 mmol/l or fasting BM >7.0 mmol/l or 2-hour BM >11.1 mmom/l after 75 g glucose tolerance test.

2 No symptoms – do not diagnose on a single glucose measurement, but do a repeat plasma test.

Patients should be classified according to pathological type (i.e. type 1 or 2) and then by stage (i.e. insulin dependent or not).

The implications of these changes are that more people will be diagnosed as being diabetic (most will be diet controlled). Hopefully, long-term complications will be reduced, but in the meantime the workload for primary care will be substantial.

Research presented at the European Association of Diabetes in September 2001 emphasised that even the new WHO guidelines on the oral glucose tolerance test (OGTT) (for those with plasma glucose 6.1–6.9 mmol/l) would miss up to 20% of people with impaired glucose tolerance, and recommended that an OGTT be performed at 5.0–6.9 mmol/l. Even by using this range, 11% of diabetes would go undetected.

National Service Framework for Diabetes (2003 Delivery Strategy)

www.doh.gov.uk/nsf/diabetes/

The document states that 'all adults with diabetes will receive high-quality care throughout their lifetime, including support to optimise the control of their blood sugar'. It includes 12 standards in nine areas of diabetic care.

1 *Prevention of type 2 diabetes*
   - Multiagency approach to reduce the number of people who are inactive, overweight and obese.
   - Physical education and a balanced diet need to be promoted from childhood.

2 *Identification of people with diabetes*
   - Follow-up of those at increased risk – gestational diabetics, known family history, ischaemic heart disease, obesity and ethnicity.

3 *Empowering people with diabetes*
   - Has been shown to reduce blood glucose and improve quality of life.
   - Could involve structured education, personal care plans and patient-held records.

4 *Clinical care of adults with diabetes*
   - Would include management of diabetes, hypertension, smoking cessation, all aimed at improving measurements and quality of life.

5 and 6 *Clinical care of children and young people with diabetes*
   - Similar high-quality care as with adults. It would also include physical, psychological, intellectual, educational and social development needs.

7 *Management of diabetic emergencies*
   - Diabetic ketoacidosis (DKA), hyperosmolar non-ketotic syndrome (HONK) and hypoglycaemia.

8 *Care of people with diabetes during admission to hospital*
   - Outcome could be improved by better liaison between diabetes team and ward staff.

9 *Diabetes and pregnancy*
- Policies will be developed for women with pre-existing diabetes and those who develop diabetes to help achieve blood pressure control before and during pregnancy.

10, 11 and 12 *Detection and management of long-term complications*
- Regular surveillance for long-term complications.
- Effective treatment and investigation for complications.
- Integrated health and social care.

Delivery strategy

- Primary care trusts will set local priorities.
- The NSF will be rolled out in conjunction with NICE guidelines.
- By 2006:
  - a minimum of 80% of diabetics should be offered screening for early detection of retinopathy (digital retinal photography)
  - this should rise to 100% by 2007
  - standards will be set by the National Screening Committee.
- Primary care priorities are as follows:
  - updating of practice registers
  - giving patients appropriate advice on diet, physical activity, smoking and treatment in line with the NSF.
- Personal diabetes record and agreed care plan include:
  - education and personal goals of the person with diabetes
  - how the diabetes will be managed until the next review and a named contact.

Effective diabetes care: a need for realistic targets
BMJ 2002; 324: 1577–80 (Education and Debate)

Aggressive treatment of hyperglycaemia, dyslipidaemia and hypertension, as well as the regular use of antiplatelet agents have been advocated in type 2 diabetes. Current targets are attainable in only 50–70% of individuals. Targets are often impractical and involve so many drugs that the patient will not comply with treatment. Individually tailored targets are needed and their effectiveness will be shown by improvement in diabetic clinics.

Training in flexible intensive insulin management to enable dietary freedom in people with type I diabetes: dose adjustments for normal eating (DAFNE) randomised controlled trial
BMJ 2002; 325: 746–9

This secondary care study from the UK looked at 169 adults with type 1 diabetes with moderate or poor glycaemic control. It was found that at 6 months the group that had been given training that promoted dietary freedom had a better quality of

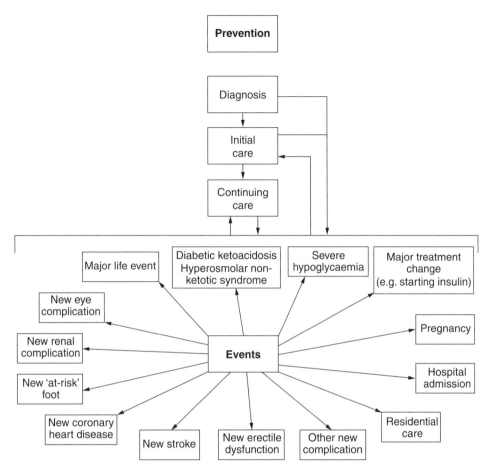

Summary of the prevention and management of diabetes.

life, better glycaemic control (HbA_{1C} mean 8.4% compared with 9.4% in non-trained) and the number of hypoglycaemic episodes was no worse.

The DAFNE programme offers a week-long intensive training course in small groups working with specialist nurses and dieticians. The course would cost £500 and is awaiting consideration by NICE.

The new treatment framework for diabetes can be summarised as follows.

1 Tools of intensive management are presented as a means to increase freedom in a patient's life.

2 The focus is on developing an insulin regimen that is flexible and fits into the demands of life.

3 The implicit message is that you can have good diabetes control without having to yield control of your life to diabetes.

NICE guidelines on the management of type 2 diabetes

Management of blood glucose levels

- HbA_{1C} should be measured 2- to 6-monthly and should be in the range 6.5–7.5%.

- Weight loss and physical activity should be encouraged if the patient is overweight.

Management of blood pressure and lipids

- An annual risk assessment should be made if there is no ischaemic heart disease. (Note that a significant number of doctors now treat cholesterol with statins, first line, despite this advice.)

- Blood pressure should be checked yearly; if >140/80 mmHg and <160/100 mmHg, recommend lifestyle changes and repeat after 6 months. If it is >140/80 mmHg and there is a high 10-year coronary risk or albuminuria, start treatment.

- Measure lipids yearly. If the cholesterol is >5 mmol/l and the triglycerides are >2.3 mmol/l, ask for advice and treat if there is an inadequate response.

$HbA_{1C} < 7.0$: what is the evidence?

Diabetes Control and Complications Trial (DCCT)

NEJM 2000; 342: 381–5 (the long-term follow-up publication)

A total of 1,441 patients were followed over a period of 6.5 years while they received either intensive treatment or conventional treatment. Intensive treatment improved microvascular and neuropathic complications, which correlates with decreased HbA_{1C} levels. The intensive treatment group did have more hypogly-caemic episodes (so would be a less favourable approach in children under 13 years and adults over 70 years).

UK Prospective Diabetes Study 33 (UKPDS 33)

Lancet 1998; 352: 837–53, 854–65

The UKPDS is a large ongoing study of type 2 diabetes involving around 5,000 patients, which was set up in 1977. It looked at newly diagnosed diabetics and treated them with diet for 3 months. If their HbA_{1C} remained elevated they were entered into the trial. It was found that intensive treatment (average HbA_{1C} 7% over the first 10 years) reduced the frequency of microvascular end points. In overweight patients with non-insulin dependent diabetes, metformin and dietary improvement reduced the risk of diabetes-related end points by 32%, and diabetic deaths by 42%. Blood pressure control (<150/85 mmHg) reduced microvascular complications and diabetic-related deaths (there were similar findings in the HOT Study, where blood pressure was reduced to <130/80 mmHg). Around 50% of diabetics had early signs of complications at the time of diagnosis (hence the importance of screening).

UKPDS 63 and 41

BMJ 2002; 325: 860–3
BMJ 2000; 320: 1373–8

These two studies concluded that the additional costs of intensive management are largely offset by significant reduction in the costs of treating complications (estimated to be £695 per patient for treatment and £957 per patient for treatment of complications, i.e. hospital admissions, outpatient visits, eye and renal problems).

UKPDS 35

BMJ 2000; 321: 405–12

Each 1% reduction in HbA_{1C} was associated with a risk reduction of 21% for diabetic end points; 21% related to diabetic deaths; 14% for myocardial infarction; and 37% for microvascular complications.

The case against aggressive treatment of type 2 diabetes: critique of UKPDS
BMJ 2001; 323: 854–8

UKPDS grew out of the author's interest in the use of basal rather than postprandial glucose. The first report was published in 1983. During the course of the study, length of follow-up has changed and end points have been redefined. The study is no longer blinded, the statistical analyses used have been questioned and the changes have not been in keeping with scientific principles.

Hypertension in diabetes

Around 70% of adults with type 2 diabetes have hypertension and more than 70% have raised cholesterol levels.

UKPDS 36 (and 49)
BMJ 2000; 321: 412–19
In type 2 diabetes the risk of diabetic complications is strongly associated with raised blood pressure. Any reduction in BP is likely to reduce the risk of complications. The lowest risk seen is in those diabetics with a systolic BP <120 mmHg. Intensive BP control is at least as important (if not more so) than intensive blood glucose control.

British Hypertension Society (BHS) guidelines based on the Hypertension Optimal Treatment Randomised Trial, 2000

- Start treatment if blood pressure is >140 mmHg systolic or >90 mmHg diastolic.

- Aim for a blood pressure 130/80 mmHg or 125/75 mmHg if there is proteinuria.

- Fewer than 30% of cases respond to monotherapy.

- *Do not forget* non-pharmacological treatment.

It is estimated that the number of diabetics on anti-hypertensives would need to double to meet targets of 140/80 mmHg.

UKPDS 36
BMJ 2000; 321: 412–19

For systolic blood pressure, each 10 mmHg decrease is associated with a risk reduction of 12% for any complications related to diabetes (15% for deaths related to diabetes, 11% for myocardial infarction and 13% for microvascular complications).

Trials

There are many more trials showing the clinical benefit of blood pressure lowering in reduction of risk (below is listed a small selection). Reference BHS, NICE and your local guidelines if you would like to look into references for a more comprehensive understanding of the trials that underpin the guidance.

● Hypertension Optimal Treatment (HOT) Randomised Trial

Effects of intensive blood pressure lowering and low-dose aspirin in patients with hypertension: principal results of the HOT trial
Lancet 1998; 351: 1755–62

The results showed low rates of cardiovascular events if raised blood pressure was lowered. There were benefits of lowering diastolic blood pressure to 82.6 mmHg, and there was a 50% decrease in major cardiovascular events with a target diastolic of 80 mmHg in diabetics compared to 90 mmHg.

Acetyl salicylic acid reduced major cardiovascular events, especially myocardial infarction. There was no effect on incidence of stroke or fatal bleeding and non-fatal major bleeds were twice as common.

● HOPE and Micro-HOPE (Health Outcome Prevention Evaluation)

Effects of ramipril on cardiovascular and microvascular outcomes in people with diabetes mellitus
Lancet 2000; 355: 253–9

A total of 3,577 diabetic patients aged 55 years and over were randomised to ramipril 10 mg/day or placebo and then vitamin E or placebo.

Ramipril had a beneficial effect on cardiovascular events, which decreased by 25–30%, and on overt nephropathy in people with diabetes. The benefit was greater than that attributable to the decrease in blood pressure. Vasculoprotective and reno-protective effects of ramipril in diabetics were seen.

Hypertension in Diabetes – targeting angiotensin
Drug Ther Bull 2005; 43(6): 41–5

This *Drugs and Therapeutics Bulletin* review gives a good overview based on weight of evidence to support treatments and may help you to develop your approach to prescribing.

Obesity in diabetes

In 1973 following research by Sims the term 'diabesity' was introduced, emphasising the link between diabetes and obesity.

Up to 80% of type 2 diabetes is due to obesity (BMI >27 kg/m^2); the duration of obesity is significant. Weight loss improves morbidity (UK Prospective Diabetes Study 7).

Diet, lifestyle and the risk of type 2 diabetes mellitus in women
NEJM 2001; 345: 790–7

A total of 84,941 female nurses aged 30–55 years were followed from 1980 to 1996. An important risk factor was a BMI >35kg/m^2. Poor diet, minimal exercise, smoking and abstinence from alcohol were all associated with significant risk of developing diabetes. It comes as no great surprise that lifestyle is a key risk.

Cholesterol and diabetes

Currently, patients with a total cholesterol >5 mmol/l or triglycerides >2.3 mmol/l with a 10-year coronary event risk >15% can be offered a statin (primary prevention). If there is already evidence of cardiovascular disease then the patient should be treated with a statin as per secondary prevention strategy (www.eguidelines.co.uk/).

The collaborative atorvastatin diabetes study: preliminary results
Int J Clin Pract 2005; 59(1): 121–3

This study looked at 2,383 40- to 45-year-old NIDDM patients with no evidence of pre-existing vascular disease. It found that 10 mg atorvastatin reduced the risk of a major cardiovascular event by 37% ($p < 0.001$) at 4 years, and the risk of stroke was almost halved. Number needed to treat to prevent 1 cardiovascular event over 4 years was 27. The trial was stopped 2 years early. The benefit of statins is thought to extend beyond LDL benefit.

Aspirin in diabetes

Given the cardiovascular risk seen in diabetes, aspirin is now considered a 'guardian drug'. Diabetes UK (www.diabetes.org.uk) recommends offering 75 mg aspirin to people over 30 years of age in the following groups of diabetic patients:

- known cardiovascular disease

- dyslipidaemia (total cholesterol >5 mmol/l)

- raised blood pressure (>140/80 mmHg) once it is controlled

- microalbuminuria or albuminuria

- family history of coronary heart disease

- smoker

- overweight (BMI $>25 \, \text{kg/m}^2$)

- Indio-Asian background

- diabetic retinopathy.

Benefit of use outside these groups is probably great, given the overall cardiovascular risk in diabetes.

Glitazones/thiazolidinediones

These drugs enhance the effects of insulin in adipose tissue and skeletal muscle by acting as ligands that regulate gene expression (i.e. they reduce the body's resistance to insulin). An increased incidence of cardiac failure has been seen with rosiglitazone when used with insulin. Pioglitazone has been licensed for use with insulin in the USA and both have been approved for monotherapy.

   Although they appear safe, it is recommended that liver function tests are performed prior to starting treatment and then at two-monthly intervals for the first year, stopping the drug if the liver enzymes rise to three times the normal level or if the patient becomes jaundiced. NICE recommends their use as second-line treatment and in combination with either metformin or a sulphonylurea.

Secondary prevention of macrovascular events in patients with type 2 diabetes in the PROACTIVE study (PROspective pioglitAzone Clinical Trial In macroVascular Events): a randomised controlled trial
Lancet **2005; 366(9493): 1241–2**

A total of 5,238 patients with type 2 diabetes and evidence of macrovascular disease (i.e. high-risk patients) were randomised to either pioglitazone or placebo. Pioglitazone improved HbA_{1C} by 0.8% (on average) and reduced all causes of mortality, non-fatal myocardial infarction and stroke.

Meglitinides/prandial glucose regulators

These are amino acid derivatives which are licensed for use with metformin in type 2 diabetes where better control is needed (i.e. $HbA_{1C} > 7.5\%$), or where patients experience hypoglycaemia when treated with sulphonylureas. The drugs are 'glucose responsive', so they induce insulin release when the patient eats, by acting on the pancreatic beta-cells to stimulate a rapid, short-lasting release of insulin to a level dependent on the glucose concentration, i.e. where there is a post-prandial rise in glucose. This is beneficial where the patient has an erratic lifestyle (e.g. junior doctors). As stimulation is not over 24 hours, the endocrine function should be preserved.

DECODE Study Group. Glucose tolerance and mortality: comparison of WHO and American Diabetes Association diagnostic criteria
Lancet **1999; 354:617–21**

This study of 18,048 men and 7,316 women aged over 30 years looked at the risk of death according to different diagnostic glucose categories, with a follow-up period of 7.3 years. It found that fasting glucose alone did not identify the risk of death associated with hyperglycaemia. Mortality increased with increasing 2-hour glucose (i.e. post-prandial spike).

Screening for diabetes

It is estimated that by 2030 half the UK population will be diabetic, and currently up to half of the people with type 2 diabetes have vascular complications at the time of diagnosis.

Mass population screening would be costly and inefficient, with a low specificity, as less than 1% of undiagnosed cases were revealed by a British Diabetic Association study in 1994. Many organisations have published arguments for a targeted approach to high-risk groups (e.g. obesity, family history of diabetes, ethnic groups, and patients with gestational diabetes, impaired glucose tolerance or hypertension).

Should we screen for type 2 diabetes? Evaluation against National Screening Committee Criteria
BMJ **2001; 322:986–8**

This discussion paper looks at the role of the National Screening Committee in evaluating a screening programme for type 2 diabetes. It summarises as follows.

- The benefits of early detection and treatment of undiagnosed diabetes have not been proved.

- The disadvantages of screening are important and should be quantified.

- Universal screening is not merited, but targeted screening may be justified.

- Clinical management of diabetes should be optimised before a screening programme is considered.

No agreement was reached on how targeted screening could be achieved. A further report is expected.

Targeting people with pre-diabetes
BMJ **2002; 325:403–4 (Editorial)**

This considers lifestyle changes and evidence that supports investment in these changes.

Diabetes UK recommends opportunistic screening for those at high risk of diabetes, and research into oral glucose tolerance testing is gradually adding weight to the argument.

Miscellaneous

Acarbose

Acarbose for prevention of type 2 diabetes mellitus: the STOP-NIDDM randomised trial
Lancet 2002; 359: 2072–7

People with impaired glucose tolerance treated with acarbose are 25% less likely to develop type 2 diabetes than those on placebo. It was concluded that acarbose could be used either as an alternative or in addition to lifestyle changes in patients with impaired glucose tolerance.

Vitamin D

Intake of vitamin D and risk of type 2 diabetes: a birth cohort study
Lancet 2001; 358: 1500–3

In this longitudinal study of 10,366 children, which was conducted between 1966 and 1997, those children who were given vitamin D (irrespective of dose) had a lower rate of type 2 diabetes. This suggests that it is important to ensure that infants get at least the recommended daily allowance of vitamin D.

Vaccine

Beta-cell function in new-onset type 1 diabetes and immunomodulation with a heat shock protein (DiaPep277): a randomised, double blind, phase III trial
Lancet 2001; 358: 1749–53

DiaPep277 is the first drug to successfully halt the immune system's destruction of pancreatic beta cells. However, the intervals at which the vaccine should be given are not known. Phase III trials are in progress.

Insulin needs after CD3 antibody therapy in new onset type 1 diabetes
NEJM 2005; 352(25): 2598–608

This study of 80 people in Belgium showed that the monoclonal antibody preserved the remaining beta-cells in newly diagnosed diabetics. Patients diagnosed early would be ideal candidates for this type of treatment – reopening the debate on the need for a screening programme.

Inhaled insulin

The first inhaled insulin to be launched is Exubera, and the UK will probably be the first country in which it is used. The inhalation into the nose delivers a dry powder to the lungs, which enables the relatively large insulin molecule to be absorbed. The role of this insulin will be similar to that of short-acting insulin. It would not be suitable for smokers, people with lung disease, women who may become pregnant or, initially, children.

Respiratory disorders

Asthma

- Around 5.4% of the population are estimated to have asthma (by National Asthma Campaign).

- New diagnoses in children rose from 4% to 10% between 1964 and 1989.

- Around 1,500 deaths per year are due to acute exacerbations of asthma.

- The annual cost of asthma to the NHS is £700 million (this does not include the economic cost of working days lost).

- Children exposed to antibiotics *in utero* are thought to be more likely to develop asthma (by up to 43%), hay fever (by up to 38%) and eczema (by up to 11%). However, this has only been shown in one study.

Historically, the second half of the twentieth century is when asthma diagnosis started to increase. Although the British Thoracic Society guidelines have been successful, asthma is still under-diagnosed and under-treated.

A recent government inquiry into asthma deaths concluded that many could have been prevented by more proactive GP care. It cited the following problems:

- under-use of primary care services
- under-prescribing of oral steroids
- inadequate use of peak expiratory flow meters (PEFR).

It also found that only 12% of those who had died had attended a practice asthma clinic in the year before death.

Some recent work has looked at the use of nitric oxide (NO), and pilot studies have found that patients with low NO levels have better asthma control and lung function.

Improvement in quality of clinical care in English general practice 1998–2003: longitudinal observational study
BMJ 2005; 331(7525): 1121

This study looked at asthma (as well as coronary heart disease and type 2 diabetes). Recording of smoking advice, peak flow and asthmatic symptoms had all improved. The score (as a measure of improvement) rose from 60.1% to 70.3% in asthma patients.

Scottish Intercollegiate Guidelines network/BTS Asthma Guidelines

Thorax **2003; 58 Suppl 1: 1–94**
www.brit-thoracic.org.uk

These guidelines, updated from the 1995 guidelines and amended in 2004, aim to achieve accurate diagnosis and symptom control quickly by stepping up treatment and then stepping down treatment when control is good.

The guidelines are broken down into adults, children aged 5–12 years and children under 5 years. They suggest that there should be a method of identifying poorly controlled asthmatics so that they can be asked to come in for review, or chased up if they fail to attend, as there is a higher mortality in this group of patients.

Step 1: short-acting bronchodilators (beta-2 agonists, ipratropium)

Step 2: introduction of a regular preventer (dose appropriate for disease severity)
There is no additional benefit in starting high and stepping down. Inhaled corticosteroids are the first choice, alternatives include:

- cromones (sodium cromoglycate)
- leukotriene-receptor antagonists
- theophyllines
- long-acting beta-2 agonists.

Step 3: add-on therapy
Long-acting beta-2 agonists are used. If the response remains suboptimal, increase the inhaled steroid dose to:

- 800 μg/day in adults
- 400 μg/day in children aged 5–12 years.

Consider further add-ons (cf. Step 2).

Step 4: addition of a fourth drug
If there is poor control on a moderate dose of inhaled steroid and add-on therapy, consider the following:

- increasing steroids to 2,000 μg/day in adults and to 800 μg/day in children aged 5–12 years
- leukotriene-receptor antagonists
- theophyllines
- slow-release beta-2 agonist tablets.

If an addition is ineffective, stop it or reduce it back to its original dose.

Step 5: continuous or frequent use of oral steroids
This is defined as either 3 months of continuous treatment or three to four courses of treatment per year.

- Immunosuppressants (methotrexate, cyclosporin and oral gold).
- Continuous subcutaneous terbutaline infusion.

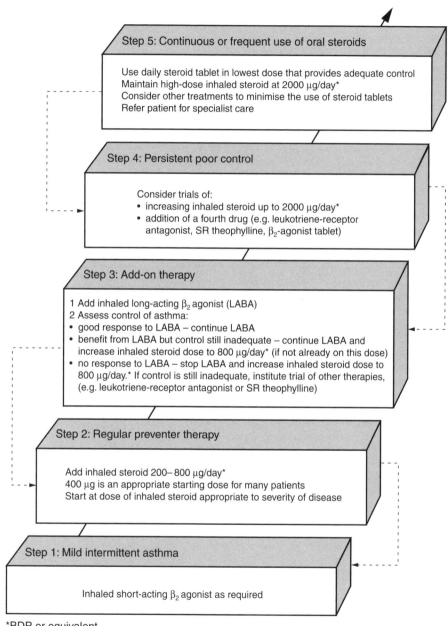

Step 5: Continuous or frequent use of oral steroids

Use daily steroid tablet in lowest dose that provides adequate control
Maintain high-dose inhaled steroid at 2000 µg/day*
Consider other treatments to minimise the use of steroid tablets
Refer patient for specialist care

Step 4: Persistent poor control

Consider trials of:
- increasing inhaled steroid up to 2000 µg/day*
- addition of a fourth drug (e.g. leukotriene-receptor antagonist, SR theophylline, β_2-agonist tablet)

Step 3: Add-on therapy

1 Add inhaled long-acting β_2 agonist (LABA)
2 Assess control of asthma:
- good response to LABA – continue LABA
- benefit from LABA but control still inadequate – continue LABA and increase inhaled steroid dose to 800 µg/day* (if not already on this dose)
- no response to LABA – stop LABA and increase inhaled steroid dose to 800 µg/day.* If control is still inadequate, institute trial of other therapies, (e.g. leukotriene-receptor antagonist or SR theophylline)

Step 2: Regular preventer therapy

Add inhaled steroid 200–800 µg/day*
400 µg is an appropriate starting dose for many patients
Start at dose of inhaled steroid appropriate to severity of disease

Step 1: Mild intermittent asthma

Inhaled short-acting β_2 agonist as required

*BDP or equivalent.

Summary of the stepwise management of asthma in adults.

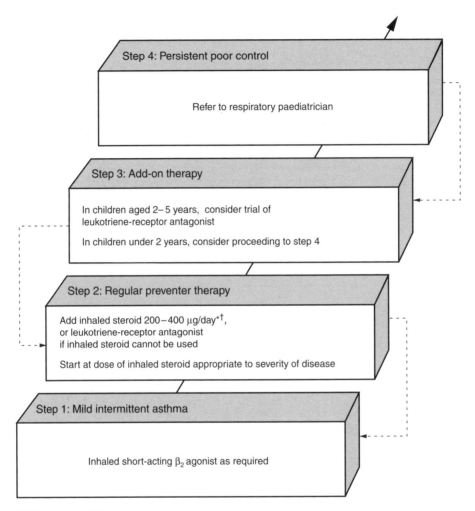

Step 4: Persistent poor control

Refer to respiratory paediatrician

Step 3: Add-on therapy

In children aged 2–5 years, consider trial of
leukotriene-receptor antagonist

In children under 2 years, consider proceeding to step 4

Step 2: Regular preventer therapy

Add inhaled steroid 200–400 μg/day*†,
or leukotriene-receptor antagonist
if inhaled steroid cannot be used

Start at dose of inhaled steroid appropriate to severity of disease

Step 1: Mild intermittent asthma

Inhaled short-acting β_2 agonist as required

*BDP or equivalent.
†Higher nominal doses may be required if drug delivery is difficult.

Summary of the stepwise management of asthma in children under 5 years of age.

Organisation of care

All practices should have a list of patients with asthma.

Review

- This should be routine with a standard recording system.
- It should include inhaler technique, PEFR, current treatment, morbidity and a personal asthma action plan (PAAP).
- It should be audited regularly.
- The best results are seen with nurses who have been trained in asthma management.

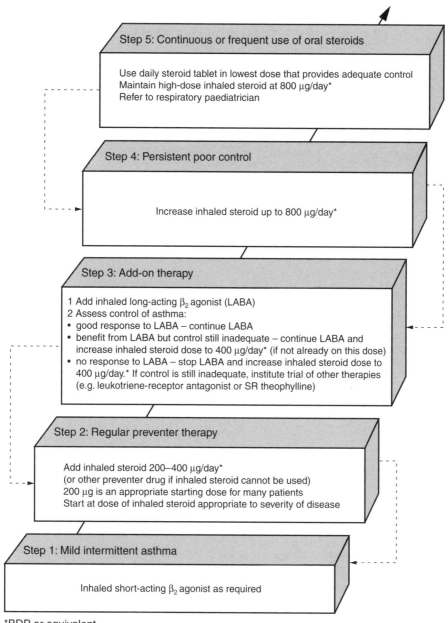

Step 5: Continuous or frequent use of oral steroids

Use daily steroid tablet in lowest dose that provides adequate control
Maintain high-dose inhaled steroid at 800 µg/day*
Refer to respiratory paediatrician

Step 4: Persistent poor control

Increase inhaled steroid up to 800 µg/day*

Step 3: Add-on therapy

1 Add inhaled long-acting β₂ agonist (LABA)
2 Assess control of asthma:
• good response to LABA – continue LABA
• benefit from LABA but control still inadequate – continue LABA and
  increase inhaled steroid dose to 400 µg/day* (if not already on this dose)
• no response to LABA – stop LABA and increase inhaled steroid dose to
  400 µg/day.* If control is still inadequate, institute trial of other therapies
  (e.g. leukotriene-receptor antagonist or SR theophylline)

Step 2: Regular preventer therapy

Add inhaled steroid 200–400 µg/day*
(or other preventer drug if inhaled steroid cannot be used)
200 µg is an appropriate starting dose for many patients
Start at dose of inhaled steroid appropriate to severity of disease

Step 1: Mild intermittent asthma

Inhaled short-acting β₂ agonist as required

*BDP or equivalent.

Summary of the stepwise management of asthma in children aged 5 to 12 years.

The following three questions should be asked.

1 Do you have difficulty sleeping because of your asthma?

2 Have you experienced your asthma symptoms during the day?

3 Has your asthma interfered with your usual activities?

Personal asthma action plans

- These should be customised and written.

- They should be offered to all patients with asthma.

Acute exacerbations

- Inpatients should be on specialist units.

- Discharge should be a planned and supervised event. It may take place as soon as clinical improvement is apparent.

Targeting care

Identify groups at risk. They include the following:

- children with frequent upper respiratory tract infections

- children over 5 years of age with persistent symptoms

- asthmatics with psychiatric disorders or learning disability

- patients who are using large quantities of beta-2 agonists.

Main additions in the 2004 update

1 Medication: inhaled steroids should be introduced in milder cases and the dose should be titrated.

2 Helping those with asthma help themselves: patients should be offered education. They should be given an individual action plan prior to hospital discharge.

3 Organisation and delivery of care: primary care services – patients should have a regular structured review.

A further addition in 2005 was the question of whether symptoms improve when the patient is away from work. If there is a suggestion of work-related asthma, patients should be referred.

Self-management plans for asthma

Since the revised 2003 BTS/SIGN guidelines, increasing importance is being placed on whether patients have the education and confidence to manage their own asthma, enabling them to live a symptom-free life by detecting and treating their exacerbations early. Personal action plans are intended for use by patients over 12 years of age.

Self-management plans reduce exacerbations, hospital admission rates and time off work, and although many asthma patients think their asthma is well managed, their symptoms (and hence quality of life) could be improved. However, the use of personal action plans is still suboptimal.

Guided self-management of asthma: how to do it
BMJ 1999; 319: 759–60 (Clinical Review)

This clinical review reached the following conclusions.

- Self-management prevents exacerbations, improves care and is cost-effective.
- Patient education is crucial and should be given in a structured way.
- Patients should be taught to understand their symptoms and monitor their PEFR at home.
- Patients should know how to act when signs of asthma deterioration first appear.
- There should always be supervision and continuity in asthma care.

Written action plans for asthma: an evidence-based review of the key components
Thorax 2004; 59(2): 94–9

This looked at 26 randomised trials and found that improved health outcomes were seen if the action plan:

- was based on a personal best peak flow reading
- used two to four action points based on symptoms or lung function
- included recommendations for inhaled and oral corticosteroid use.

Long-acting beta-2 agonists

MIASMA (meta-analysis of increased dose of inhaled steroid or addition of salmeterol in symptomatic asthma)
BMJ 2000; 320: 1368–73

Lung function was higher in patients who received salmeterol rather than steroids. Symptom-free days and nights were more frequent with salmeterol, as were rescue-free days and nights. There was less exacerbation of symptoms with salmeterol, and the severity was less in those who did experience this.

Leukotriene-receptor antagonists

These are derived from arachidonic acid, the precursor of prostaglandins. By preventing prostaglandin release, they reduce bronchoconstriction, mucus secretion and oedema.

Randomised controlled trial of montelukast plus inhaled budesonide versus double dose of inhaled budesonide in adult patients with asthma
Thorax **2003; 58: 211–16**
This multinational trial compared the addition of montelukast 10 mg/day to doubling the steroid dose in 889 adults with asthma. Lung function improved earlier with montelukast, but after 6 weeks both strategies had worked.

Improving asthma control in patients suboptimally controlled on inhaled corticosteroids and long-acting beta-2 agonists: addition of montelukast in an open label pilot study
Curr Med Res Opin **2005; 21(6): 863–9**

This is a real-life observational study of 313 patients in Belgium already taking inhaled corticosteroids and long-acting beta-2 agonists, but who were inadequately controlled. It found that 78.6% of the patients reported an improvement in their asthma with the addition of montelukast.

Chlorofluorocarbon (CFC)-free inhalers

- CFCs have implications for the depletion of the ozone layer.

- They can be used as propellants in metered-dose inhalers (MDIs).

- CFC-free MDIs have been available since 1995 in the UK and are now being widely used.

- Hydrofluoroalkane (HFA) compounds are being used in preference; their safety profile is similar to CFCs.

Breathing exercises

The Butekyo method is a breathing technique developed by a Russian physician who believes that a significant amount of asthma is caused by hyperventilation. In the UK, this can be taught by a trained physiotherapist.

As yet there is no reliable body of evidence to indicate whether breathing exercises work to reduce symptoms of asthma (Cochrane Review, 2001), although it would make sense if they did.

The use of tumour necrosis factors (TNF) blockers is being trialled, alongside usual treatment, for brittle asthmatics. Also under consideration is an injection of omalizumab (a protein that blocks the immune response to allergens), which could prevent severe allergy-related asthma attacks. It would be administered by injection every 2 to 4 weeks.

Chronic obstructive pulmonary/airways disease

Chronic obstructive pulmonary disease (COPD) has recently been recognised as a systemic disease. The systemic symptoms of muscle weakness and weight loss seem to relate poorly to lung function, hence lung function should be only one of the tools we use to assess disease severity and progression.

British Thoracic Society (BTS) definition

'A chronic slowly progressive disorder characterised by airflow obstruction that does not change markedly over several months. Most of the lung function is fixed, although some reversibility can be produced by bronchodilator (or other) therapy.'

- COPD causes around 26,000 deaths per year (respiratory disease is now the biggest killer in the UK).

- It is responsible for 400–1,000 per 10,000 consultations in general practice.

- Risk factors include smoking, pollution, occupation (cadmium and coal related), lower social classes, genetic factors and chronic under-treatment of asthma.

The BTS published guidelines in 1997 aimed at improving diagnosis and management (*Thorax* **1997; 52 Suppl 5: S1–28**). GOLD has also published COPD guidelines at www.goldcopd.com.

It is thought (following a recent publication in *Chest* **2005; October**) that the UK BTS guidelines may miss 1.5% cases of COPD when compared with the use of the European Respiratory Society guidelines (the difference being that BTS guidelines are fixed and ERS guidelines are weighted for gender).

NICE Chronic obstructive pulmonary disease February 2004

This is available for reference, and the summary is probably more concise than the BTS guidelines for ease of everyday use.

Diagnosis of COPD

This is suggested by symptoms and established by objective measurements using spirometry, with a chest X-ray to exclude other pathologies.

Spirometry is the most reliable means of confirming a diagnosis and assessing severity and reversibility. A trial of steroids (30 mg prednisolone for 2 weeks, or 6 weeks of beclomethasone 1,000 μg per day), following baseline spirometry, is recommended when looking for reversibility. Reversibility is an increase of FEV_1 by 15% *and* 200 ml above the baseline.

In October 2001, *GP News* looked at the potential savings that could be made by identifying COPD patients on asthma registers and withdrawing inhaled steroids (following data presented at the 11th European Respiratory Society Conference).

An observational study of inhaled corticosteroid withdrawal in stable COPD
Resp Med **1999; 93: 161–6**

This study pointed out the risk of exacerbation in stopping inhaled corticosteroids, and advocated careful monitoring.

Steroid use in COPD

Inhaled corticosteroids and mortality in COPD
Thorax 2005; 60: 992–7

Studies suggest that corticosteroids reduce exacerbations and improve health status in COPD. This analysis pooled seven randomised trials (5,085 patients) to look at mortality. It found that inhaled corticosteroids reduced all causes of mortality in COPD by up to 27%, during a mean follow-up of 26 months.

TRISTAN (Trial of inhaled steroids and long-acting beta-2 agonists)
Lancet 2003; 361: 449–56

In this trial of 1,465 patients, after 12 months of combined treatment (salmeterol and fluticasone) there was a significantly greater improvement in lung function than with either monotherapy or placebo. Combined therapy was also associated with the greatest reduction in symptoms.

There is growing evidence that oral steroids help reduce exacerbations (Cochrane Review, 2001). One randomised controlled trial showed that a 10-day course of steroids was better than a 3-day course. One review suggested that oral steroids decreased the length of hospital stay by 1–2 days, and this was not at the expense of raised blood sugars or secondary infections.

Smoking cessation

This reduces the rate of decline in lung function (***BMJ* 1977; 1: 1645–8.** *See* graph below, and also section on smoking cessation, p. 22 *et seq.*).

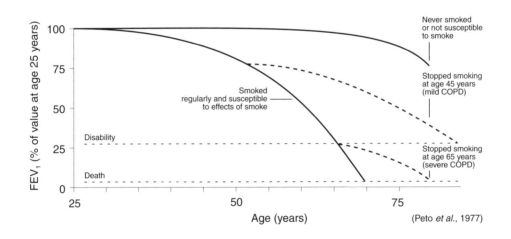

Environmental tobacco smoke and risk of respiratory cancer and chronic obstructive pulmonary disease in former smokers and never smokers in the EPIC prospective study
BMJ **2005; 330: 277–80**

This was a prospective study of 303,020 people who had never smoked or who had stopped smoking at least 10 years previously, and who provided information about environmental tobacco smoke. Controls were matched for sex, age, smoking status and country of recruitment. Over a 7-year follow-up period the whole cohort had an increased risk of events (hazard ratio 1.30, 95% CI 0.87–1.95). The study concluded that environmental tobacco smoke was a risk factor for respiratory diseases, especially in ex-smokers.

Long-term oxygen therapy (LTOT)

In hypoxaemic patients, LTOT prolongs life.

Patients with cyanosis and cor pulmonale should be considered for LTOT assessment. LTOT should be considered if PaO_2 <7.3 kPa, but it is important to ensure that it does not cause carbon dioxide retention. Oxygen should be prescribed for 15–20 hours per day.

MRC Trial
Lancet **1981; 1 (8222): 681–6**

This trial showed that five patients would need to be treated for 5 years to avoid one death (i.e. NNT = 5), where treatment involved administration of oxygen for 15 hours per day. The difference was only evident after 500 hours.

Domiciliary oxygen for COPD
Cochrane Database Syst Review **2005 Oct 19; 4: CD001744**

Six randomised controlled trials were identified. Long-term oxygen therapy improved survival of patients with severe hypoxaemia (arterial PaO_2 <55 mmHg [8.0 kPa]).

Self-management plans for COPD

The principles follow the same lines as those for asthma management plans.

Self-management reduces both short- and long-term hospitalisation in COPD
Eur Resp J **2005; 26(5): 853–7**

This Canadian study involving 191 patients who had been hospitalised with an exacerbation of their COPD involved a randomised issuing of the self-management programme 'Living with COPD' versus standard hospital care. At 2 years the intervention group showed a reduction from 26.9% to 21.1% cases of hospitalisation.

Action plans for COPD

Cochrane Database Syst Review **2005 Oct 19; 4: CD005074**

The review showed that action plans helped patients to recognise symptoms of an exacerbation and helped them to self-initiate antibiotics or oral steroids successfully.

N-acetylcysteine

This is a mucolytic agent with anti-oxidant properties that has been found to reduce the exacerbations of COPD (NNT = 6). It may also slow the rate of decline in lung function.

New developments in the treatment of COPD: comparing the effects of inhaled corticosteroids and N-acetylcysteine
J Physiol Pharmacol **2005; 56 Suppl 4: 135–42**

The results of this complicated study showed that inhaled corticosteroids improved lung function in COPD. The N-acetylcysteine group showed a reduction in inflammatory markers.

Pulmonary rehabilitation

This has been shown to reduce symptoms, increase mobility and improve quality of life. It will become an increasing part of the holistic care approach we should have as GPs.

   Exercise can reduce the risk of relapses that require hospital admission by 50% (*Thorax* **2003; 58: 100–5**).

Pulmonary rehabilitation and the BODE index in COPD
Eur Resp J **2005; 26(4): 630–6**

The BODE index integrates body mass index, airflow limitation (forced expiratory volume in 1 second), dyspnoea and a 6-minute walking distance. It predicts mortality in COPD. A total of 246 patients were divided into groups of patients who had received pulmonary rehabilitation and those who had not. BODE worsened by 4% over 12 months in those with no rehabilitation, mortality in this group was 39%. BODE improved by 19% following rehabilitation, but returned to the original baseline after 2 years, mortality in this group was 7%. It is thought that the BODE index change after pulmonary rehabilitation may provide valuable prognostic information.

Long-acting anticholinergics

Tiotropium is a once-daily maintenance dose for COPD that has been shown to improve FEV_1 against placebo, salmeterol and ipratropium.

Prevention of exacerbation of COPD with tiotropium, a once-daily inhaled anticholinergic bronchodilator: a randomized trial
Ann Intern Med 2005; 143(5): 317–26

This was an American study of 1,829 patients with moderate to severe COPD. Tiotropium, after 6 months' use, was found to reduce exacerbations (there were 27.9% compared with 32.3% in the placebo group).

Osteoporosis

There is a higher risk of osteoporosis in COPD (compared with asthma), even when patients have not had long-term steroid treatment (*Chest* 2003; 122: 1949–55). The cause of this is not completely understood, although the multisystemic effects, poor nutrition and lower testosterone levels probably all contribute to the effect.

Influenza

It is estimated that, in the UK, flu causes 2,000–4,000 deaths per year, mainly between December and March. In America, it is known that 10–20% of the population will show serological conversion, whether or not they are symptomatic, each year.

Immunisation

Immunisation of those at high risk of serious illness from influenza reduces hospital admissions and deaths. Immunisation can reduce mortality by up to 40% (up to 70% in repeated vaccination) and respiratory illness by up to 50%.

In October every year there is a fantastic influenza immunisation campaign run by primary care, which aims to reduce morbidity and mortality. Currently, work is looking into children and their role in transmission of the virus, as well as how the illness affects them. They may be part of new inclusion groups in future campaigns, which are sent out yearly by the Chief Medical Officer (CMO).

The Department of Health's flu campaign targets all people over 65 years and all people over 6 months of age in the following risk groups:

- all high-risk groups (cardiovascular disease, diabetes, immunosuppression and chronic diseases, including chronic liver disease)

- all those in long-stay residential and nursing homes, as well as other long-stay facilities

- people who are the main carer for an elderly or disabled person, whose welfare may be at risk if their carer falls ill (added 2005).

CMO immunisation programme 2005 targets
- A minimum target of 70% in those over 65 years of age. The World Health Organization has set targets of 85% to be achieved by 2010 (alongside this the GP contract sets out percentages that need to be achieved in certain disease areas).

- NHS employers should offer the vaccination to employees directly involved in patient care through the occupational health service, not their own GPs (unless they have been specifically contracted). Vaccines for staff should not be obtained at the expense of vaccine for the high-risk groups.

A number of different articles in the *British Journal of General Practice* found variously that patients who decline flu vaccine:

- consider influenza a mild disease

- hope they won't get flu

- doubt the effectiveness of the vaccine

- fear the side effects of the vaccine and that it will give them flu

- lack campaign awareness

- are apathetic

- are unable to attend for immunisation (e.g. because they are housebound or in residential care)

- find the timing of immunisation clinics inconvenient

- lack information about the vaccination.

Influenza immunization uptake and distribution in England and Wales using data from the general practice research database 1989/90–2003/04
J Public Health 2005; Oct 5

Major changes to the influenza vaccination programme were introduced in 1998 and 2000 (immunisation of elderly patients became age-related rather than risk-related). This review examined groups by age and medical risk. Vaccine uptake among high-risk individuals over 65 years of age increased from 36.7% in 1989/90 to 72.1% in 2003/04. Vaccine uptake among high-risk individuals under 65 years increased from 10.8% in 1989/90 to 24.3% in 2003/04. This is still well below satisfactory levels, and it will be interesting to see the follow-through from implementation of the new contract.

Pneumococcal vaccine
This is a one-off vaccination (revaccinate after 5–10 years if antibody levels are likely to have declined). It can be given at the same time as the influenza vaccination, but at different sites.

The Department of Health Pneumococcal Immunization Programme was introduced in August 2003 as an all-year-round campaign. The age of eligibility for vaccination has gradually been reduced. Current target groups (April 2005) include:

- all people over 65 years

- at-risk groups, from the age of 2 months (the main difference to the flu programme is that asthma is not included unless the patient needs frequent oral corticosteroids)

- individuals with cochlear implants

- individuals with the potential for cerebrospinal fluid leaks

- children under 5 years who have had a previously invasive pneumococcal disease.

Antiretroviral treatment for influenza

The neuraminidase inhibitors inhibit the replication of influenza A and B. They should be started within 48 hours of symptoms developing and are designed to complement the vaccination programme. Amantidine has been available since the 1970s, but is only effective against influenza A. If there is an influenza pandemic, of whatever strain, these drugs will be part of our management. It is not yet clear if they have a significant role to play in prophylaxis.

NICE 58 (February 2003) Guidance on the use of zanamivir, oseltamivir and amantidine

This states that these should be used if influenza A or B is circulating in the community, and also in at-risk groups, namely those with chronic respiratory or renal disease, significant cardiovascular disease (not hypertension) or diabetes, and those who are immunocompromised or over 65 years of age.

Oseltamivir in the management of influenza
Expert Opin Pharmacother 2005; 6(14): 2493–500

A worldwide flu pandemic could cause 20–40 million deaths. This report summarises that the World Health Organization has recommended stockpiling oseltamivir for such an occasion, as it not only reduces the severity and duration of symptoms, complications and mortality, but has also been shown to be effective against the circulating strain H5N1 (bird flu).

Health Technology Assessment Report (December 2000)

This meta-analysis of six randomised controlled trials (not brilliant trials, as risk groups formed small minorities) included 800 at-risk patients. The duration of influenza symptoms was reduced by 1.2 days (95% CI, 0.1–2.2), from 6 to 5 days, if Relenza was used. Relenza also reduced the risk of complications requiring antibiotics. No data on hospitalisation were provided.

Comparison of elderly people's technique in using two dry powder inhalers to deliver zanamivir: randomised controlled trial
BMJ 2001; 322: 577–9

Delivery of zanamivir was as a dry powder through a Diskhaler. The study concluded that most elderly people (i.e. one cohort deemed to be at high risk) were unable to use the inhaler device, so treatment with the drug was unlikely to be effective unless this delivery system could be improved.

Women's health

Hormone replacement therapy (HRT)

This is a collective term to encompass a variety of sex steroids, oestrogens and progesterones given in various forms. Treatment with HRT is a curious ethical problem and is always topical.

Menopause in the UK usually occurs around the age of 51 years. Our current target population of women who should be given the opportunity to make an informed decision on whether or not to take HRT includes the following:

- women with menopausal symptoms affecting their quality of life (usually short-term use)

- women who have had a premature menopause (under the age of 40 years)

- women who have had a surgical menopause (hysterectomy and oophorectomy) under the age of 40 years. Use of HRT in this group is usually until the age menopause would have occurred.

Managing the menopause – British Menopause Society Council Consensus Statement on HRT, 10 June 2005

This concludes that results from recent papers have thus far given no reason to make any changes in current clinical practice. Below is a brief summary of the statement.

Benefits

1 *Vasomotor symptoms* – there is good evidence from randomised controlled trials (RCT), with improvement usually noted within 4 weeks.

2 *Urogenital symptoms and sexuality symptoms* – these respond well to oestrogens (topically or systemically). Long-term treatment is often needed.

3 *Osteoporosis* – there is evidence from RCTs (including the Women's Health Initiative (WHI) and the Million Women Study) that HRT reduces hip as well as other osteoporotic fractures. It is not advised that HRT be used as first-line treatment for prevention of osteoporosis. Benefit wears off rapidly after cessation of use.

4 *Colorectal cancer* – results from the oestrogen progestogen arm (WHI) only shows that HRT reduces the risk of colorectal cancer. It is not advised that HRT be used for prevention.

Risks

1 *Breast cancer* – mammographic density is increased in about 25% of women. HRT appears to confer a similar degree of risk as that associated with a late natural menopause (2.3% compared with 2.8% per year respectively). The lifetime risk is significantly increased with current long-term use when started over the age of 50 years (relative risk of 1.35, 95% CI 1.2–1.49). Such an effect is not seen in women who start HRT for a premature menopause, indicating that it is the duration of lifetime hormone exposure that is relevant. Progesterone addition

increases the risk of breast cancer and has to be balanced against the fact that if not used, the risk of endometrial cancer will increase. Breast cancer risk falls after cessation of use, and by 5 years is no greater than if never exposed to HRT.

2 *Endometrial cancer* – unopposed oestrogen increases endometrial cancer. Sequential progesterone does not eliminate this risk.

3 *Venous thromboembolism* – HRT increases the risk twofold, the highest risk being in the first year of use. Absolute risk is small at 1.7 per 1,000 in women over 50 years of age.

4 *Gallbladder disease* – HRT increases the risk (confirmed in the WHI).

Uncertainties

1 *Cardiovascular disease* – the role of HRT for primary and secondary prevention remains uncertain. The WHI showed a transient increase in coronary heart disease; absolute risk at 50–59 years was 5, and at 60–69 years was 1.

2 *Dementia and cognition* – while oestrogen may delay or reduce the risk of Alzheimer's disease, it does not seem to improve established disease.

3 *Ovarian cancer* – in oestrogen-only, after more than 10 years of use there seems to be an increase in the risk. In continuous combined therapy this does not seem to be the case.

4 *Quality of life* – this is difficult to evaluate, and there is no conclusion as yet.

Women's Health Initiative

This was two separate, parallel, multicentre, randomised, double blind, placebo controlled studies evaluating the risks and benefits of conjugated equine oestrogen both alone and in combination with medroxyprogesterone acetate in healthy postmenopausal women.

It looked at 16,608 postmenopausal women with an intact uterus (there was a further arm of 10,739 patients who had previously undergone a hysterectomy), aged 50–79 years from September 1993 to July 2002. Participants were randomly assigned to either conjugated equine oestrogens (0.625 mg per day) or conjugated equine oestrogens (0.625 mg per day) plus medroxyprogesterone acetate (2.5 mg per day). The women were followed up for a mean of 5.2 years. Results were published over several papers (mainly in *JAMA*), and the main findings were as follows:

• HRT does not confer cardiovascular or cognitive protection

• HRT increases the risk of breast cancer in women with a uterus

• HRT increases the risk of venothromboembolism

• HRT does not improve overall quality of life

• HRT reduces fracture rates

• HRT reduces vasomotor symptoms.

There are many facets to this trial (for example breast cancer risk is further broken down into association with obesity, exercise and use of non-steroidal anti-inflammatories – all in separate articles). The latest article (*JAMA* **2005; 293: 935–48**) shows that HRT worsens urinary incontinence, where it had previously been thought to improve it.

Estrogen plus progestin and the risk of coronary heart disease
NEJM **2003; 349(6): 523–34**

The primary efficacy outcome of the trial was CHD (non-fatal myocardial infarction or death due to CHD). Termination of the study was advised after a mean of 5.2 years' follow-up. The elevation in risk was most apparent in the combined hormone therapy group at 1 year (hazard ratio 1.81; 95% CI 1.09–3.01), but overall it was found to have an associated hazard ratio of 1.24 (95% CI 1.00–1.54, 95% CI after adjustment for sequential monitoring 0.97–1.60).

Criticism related to the WHI Study
This is a general collection of thoughts from many authors across many publications and is by no means exhaustive.

- A high dose of conjugated equine oestrogens was the choice for HRT.

- Women were, on average, 63 years at the start of treatment (most women who use HRT are between the ages of 45 and 55 years and are symptomatic).

- It looked at post-menopausal women so cannot be extrapolated to women with an early menopause.

- Women taking HRT in the UK are a self-selecting group, usually educated and in a high socioeconomic class, with a better diet, and are less likely to come from ethnic minority backgrounds (the trial included all women).

- There is a danger that trials that are stopped early are at a random high, it is important to be cautious about fast-tracking results into practice.

WHI Clinical trial revisit: imprecise scientific methodology disqualifies the study's outcomes
Am J Obstet Gynecol **2005; 193(5): 1599–604**

This is a discussion paper about the lack of independent, non-biased analysis of the quality of methodology. The authors feel that the questions over the study's validity make it difficult to apply the WHI results to healthy post-menopausal women, different ethnic groups or as general post-menopausal prevention.

Assessment of the understanding of the risks and benefits of HRT in primary care physicians
Am J Obstet Gynecol **2005; 193(2): 551–6**

In this study, 600 returned questionnaires from Florida found that following the WHI, although gynaecologists had a better understanding, respondents overestimated risk by confusing relative risk with absolute risk.

The Million Women Study

Breast cancer and HRT in the Million Women Study
Lancet 2003; 362(9382): 419–27

This is an observational study that was set up to investigate the effects of specific types of HRT on incident and fatal breast cancer. A total of 1,084,110 women living in the UK and aged between 50 and 64 years were recruited between 1996 and 2001. They provided information about their use of HRT and other personal details and were followed up for cancer incidence and death. The study found that current users of HRT were more likely than never users to develop breast cancer (relative risk 1.66; 95% CI 1.58–1.75; $p < 0.0001$) and die from it (relative risk 1.22; 95% CI 1.00–1.48; $p = 0.05$). Past users were not at increased risk. The associated risk was greater for oestrogen–progestogen than other forms of HRT ($p < 0.0001$), and the risk varied little between the strength and type of HRT.

HRT and stroke: clinical trials review
Stroke 2004; 35(11 Suppl 1): 2644–7

Observational data suggest that postmenopausal HRT is associated with a 25–50% lower cardiovascular disease. However, observational data for HRT are associated with the potential for bias.

Of the three major trials on stroke and postmenopausal women, two focus on secondary prevention:

- the Heart and Estrogen/progestin Replacement Study (HERS)
- Women's Estrogen for Stroke Trial (WEST)

and one examined primary prevention:

- the Women's Health Initiative (WHI).

All indicate that postmenopausal hormone therapy is not effective at reducing stroke, either in established vascular disease or as primary prevention.

Association between HRT and subsequent stroke: a meta-analysis
BMJ 2005; 330: 342–5

This analysis looked at 28 trials with 39,769 subjects. It found that HRT was associated with increased incidence of stroke, particularly of ischaemic type. Of the people who had a stroke, those taking HRT seemed to have a worse outcome.

Alternatives to HRT

For hot flushes

The research base for these products is limited, although undoubtedly some women get very real relief from these products.

- Phyto-oestrogens (found in chickpeas, lentils, soya products, red clover) – there have been several small randomised controlled trials comparing, for example, soy flour to wheat flour. They have found no significant reduction in hot flushes.

- Black cohosh – a recent study in *Maturitas* (**2005; 16: 134–46**) found that it offered no significant benefit.

- Dong quai.

- Evening primrose oil.

- *Ginkgo biloba.*

- Clonidine (an alpha adrenoceptor agonist).

- Selective serotonin reuptake inhibitors.

- Acupuncture (usually a small tack left in at the ankle that can be massaged).

For osteoporosis

- Bisphosphonates, e.g. aledronate, etidronate, residronate.

- Strontium ranelate.

For mood disturbances

- St John's Wort.

- Antidepressant medication.

Menorrhagia

Menorrhagia is the loss of >80 ml of blood per cycle (with either regular or irregular cycles). It is important to assess the condition properly for primary and secondary causes.

- Around 28% of women feel menstruation is excessive and 5% consult their GP.

- One in 20 women aged 30–49 years consult their GP each year with menorrhagia.

- One in five women will have a hysterectomy before the age of 60 years.

- GPs should focus on quality of life issues.

The Royal College of Obstetricians and Gynaecologists current evidence-based guidelines are in favour of using tranexamic acid with or without mefanamic acid to reduce blood loss. They do not recommend routine thyroid function tests unless there are other suggestive symptoms.

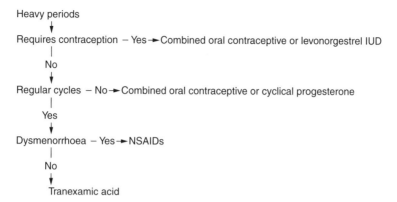

Heavy periods
↓
Requires contraception − Yes → Combined oral contraceptive or levonorgestrel IUD
|
No
↓
Regular cycles − No → Combined oral contraceptive or cyclical progesterone
|
Yes
↓
Dysmenorrhoea − Yes → NSAIDs
|
No
↓
Tranexamic acid

Pre-menstrual syndrome

This is a distinct disorder (of emotional and physical symptoms) that occurs in the luteal phase of the cycle due to the release of progesterone triggered by ovulation. There is no evidence of a specific hormonal imbalance. Meta-analyses have confirmed that treatment with progesterone products is no more effective than placebo.

There is no diagnostic test. The best way to diagnose premenstrual syndrome (PMS) is by asking the patient to keep a 3-month diary which should show cyclical premenstrual deterioration with postmenstrual cure.

Treatment

There are two broad approaches.

Suppressing ovulation
- Combined oral contraceptive pill (variable response).

- Danazol (several randomised controlled trials prove benefit, although the long-term use is limited due to masculinising effects).

- Oestrogen patches or implants − progestogenic endometrial protection (e.g. Mirena) is needed, as well as assessment of the endometrium at the outset of treatment so as not to risk falsely reassuring a woman that bleeding is normal when she may indeed have endometrial cancer.

- Gonadotrophin-releasing hormones (pharmacological menopause − time limited unless add-back HRT or tibolone is used).

- Oophorectomy and hysterectomy (rarely justified).

Changing serotonin status
- Vitamin B_6 (50–100 mg maximum, as there is a risk of peripheral neuropathy) has been shown to give some improvement. Vitamin E may be of benefit in breast tenderness.

- Selective serotonin reuptake inhibitors (SSRIs) appear to be seven times more effective than placebo but must not be prescribed with St John's Wort.

Luteal phase dosing with paroxetine controlled release in the treatment of premenstrual dysmorphic disorder
Am J Obstet Gynecol **2005; 193(2): 352–60**

This multicentre randomised double-blind placebo-controlled trial looked at either 12.5 mg or 25 mg of paroxetine daily in the luteal phase versus placebo (in a total of 373 patients). Both doses were found to be effective, well tolerated and significantly better than placebo.

Other treatment options

- *Agnus castus fruit extract*: this fruit from the Chast tree has been a traditional remedy for PMS.

  Treatment for PMS with agnus castus fruit extract: prospective, randomised, placebo-controlled trial
  BMJ **2001; 322(7279): 134–7**

  A total of 178 German women were randomised for three cycles. Agnus castus fruit was found to be significantly more effective than placebo, and it appears to be safe.

- *St John's Wort*: initial studies have shown a possible benefit. It does help depressive features irrespective of other symptoms.

- *Dietary changes* such as increasing soy isoflavins have been seen to give some improvement.

- *Complementary therapies*:
  - acupuncture has been shown to help features of dysmenorrhoea
  - homeopathy has been found in a pilot study of 20 women to produce a 90% improvement compared with placebo
  - Qi therapy, aromatherapy, reflexology, photic stimulation and magnetic therapy all have some supporting anecdotal evidence.

Contraception

The global population is estimated to reach 8.9 billion by 2050, and with it come significant risks of over-population. The goals of contraception are ultimately to reduce the number of unplanned and unwanted pregnancies by safe, well-tolerated and reversible methods.

Hormonal methods of contraception have been slow to change over the past four decades due to social, political and legal reasons, as well as medical complications encountered.

Combined oral contraception

In the UK, 25% of women aged 16–49 years and 50% of women in their twenties are on the pill. Currently, all pharmacological methods of contraception are reversible and made from synthetic steroids, containing no natural oestrogens or progesterones.

There are three generations of combined pill.

1 First generation (e.g. Norinyl-1, Ovran):
   - first produced in the 1960s
   - high dose of oestrogen (increased veno-thromboembolism (VTE) risk)
   - avoided now unless specifically needed (e.g. with enzyme-inducing drugs such as anti-epileptics).

2 Second generation:
   - lower oestrogen
   - similar progestogen to first-generation pill.

3 Third generation:
   - produced in the 1980s
   - lower dose of oestrogen
   - new form of progestogen (less androgenic than second-generation products)
   - 1995 pill scare – the Committee on Safety of Medicines stated that VTE risk was doubled in users of pills that contained gestodene or desogestrel. This was based on unpublished trials with no confidence intervals. It was the first time progestogens had been implicated.

Risk assessment
It is important to assess risk before initiating treatment and at each review.

- VTE risk increases with increasing age.

- BMI $>35\,kg/m^2$ quadruples the risk of VTE. There are other alternatives, so use them if you possibly can.

- Smoking doubles the risk of VTE.

- Family history – if patients have a first-degree relative under 45 years of age with VTE/primary thrombotic tendency, then combined pills should not be used.

- Ask about migraines (focal), breast cancer, pregnancy, undiagnosed vaginal bleed and diabetes.

- Measure blood pressure.

Veno-thromboembolism
In 1 year:

- 5 in 100,000 women will develop VTE

- 15 in 100,000 will develop VTE if taking second-generation pill (levonorgestrel/ norethisterone)

- 25 in 100,000 will develop VTE if taking third-generation pill (gestodene/ desogestrel)

- 60 in 100,000 will develop VTE in pregnancy.

The absolute risk, as opposed to the relative risk, is small. If after 1 year of pill use a woman has not experienced a clot, it is thought that the subsequent risk will then be much lower.

Since the 1980s, the accepted risk for VTE due to combined oral contraceptives has been 30 in 100,000. Therefore, studies did not necessarily suggest an increased risk in third-generation pills but a reduced risk, and a higher risk with second-generation pills than originally thought.

In 1999, the Department of Health announced an end to the 1995 restrictions on prescribing third-generation pills.

UK studies
Third-generation oral contraceptives and the risk of venous thrombosis: meta-analysis
BMJ 2001; 323: 131–4

This meta-analysis supports the view that third-generation pills have a greater risk than second generation pills with regard to venous thrombosis. The overall adjusted odds ratio was 1.7 (95% CI 1.4–2.0). The nine case-control studies looked at patients who had had a thrombosis and whether they used the oral contraceptive pill. This does not prove that the pill caused the clots.

Mortality associated with oral contraceptive use: 25-year follow-up of 46,000 women from RCGP oral contraceptive study
BMJ 1999; 318: 96–100

Among a total of 1,599 deaths reported from 1,400 practices in the UK, 945 deaths were of women who had at some time used the pill and 654 deaths were of never-users. The death rate from all causes combined was 21% lower than in the UK population (for age). This finding was not unexpected, as women with severe chronic illnesses were excluded. Most of the effects on mortality occurred in current or recent users, and few if any effects persisted 10 years after stopping use of the pill.

The study confirmed the following.

- The risk of breast cancer is slightly increased, but there is no excess risk after stopping for 10 years.

- The risk of cervical cancer is increased, but there seems to be no excess risk after stopping for 10 years. There is a question as to whether the combined pill potentiates human papillomavirus rather than the increase reflecting promiscuity.

- The risk of circulatory disease is increased in users/recent users of the pill.

- The risk of ovarian cancer is reduced in users/recent users of the pill.

Oral contraceptives and the risk of breast cancer
NEJM 2002; 346: 2025–32

This was a population-based, case-controlled study (4,575 women with breast cancer and 4,682 controls were interviewed). The relative risk of developing breast cancer having taken the pill was 1.0 (95% CI 0.8–1.0).

Combined oral contraceptives and cervical cancer
Curr Opin Obstet Gynecol 2004; 16(1): 27–9

This was a literature review that included eight studies conducted by the International Agency for Research on Cancer. The epidemiological links suggest an increased risk of cervical cancer (up to twofold) but only for women who are long-term users (5 years or more) and who have persistent human papillomavirus infections of the cervix.

Long-acting reversible contraceptives (LARCs)

NICE October 2005
NICE starts by saying that the profession should take into account women's individual needs and preferences. The following recommendations have been identified as priorities.

1 Contraceptive provision:
   - information and choice of all methods of contraception should be offered
   - contraceptive service providers should be aware that all currently available LARC methods (IUDs, IUS, injectables and implants) are more cost-effective than the pill at 1 year. IUDs, IUS and implants are more cost-effective than injectables, and increasing the use of LARCs will reduce the risk of pregnancy.

2 Counselling and provision of information:
   - should be both written and verbal and include: efficacy of method, duration of use, risk and possible side effects, non-contraceptive benefits, procedure for initiation and discontinuation, and when to seek help while using the method
   - should include advice on safer sex.

Implanon
This was launched in September 1999 (following the withdrawal of Norplant because of problems relating to the insertion and removal of six rods). It consists of a single semi-rigid rod with dimensions of 40 mm × 2 mm. Insertion should be performed subdermally, and the device releases 30–40 μg etonogestrel/day. It lasts for a total of 3 years and has a Pearl Index of 0.

Amenorrhoea is reported in around 21% of women and irregular bleeding can be problematic (as expected with progesterone methods) in around 17% of women, although by 6 months this has often settled.

There have been reports of fractures of the implant following minor trauma, and there has been one report of a pregnancy after 18 months in a woman on anti-epileptic medication.

Coils
1 Copper coils (380 mm copper) are relatively easy to insert, even in nulliparous women. The licence is usually from 8–10 years, depending on the type of coil and the time of insertion related to the menopause. The failure rate at 2 years is around 1.6 per 100 women (60% were due to expulsion). At least 300 mm of copper is needed for contraception to be effective.

2 Mirena is licensed for 5 years only (even if fitted in women over 40 years), although it is probably OK for 7 years. The NICE guidelines state that if the woman is ammenorrhoeic it is fine to keep the IUS *in situ* until it is no longer needed for contraception (not as straightforward as it might seem, given that the need for contraception is usually based on having stopped menses with no hormonal influence).

3 Gynaefix is a frameless IUD consisting of six copper tubes on a nylon thread, knotted at one end, which anchors into the uterine fundus. The failure rate is less than 1% in up to 5 years of use and the expulsion rate is low.

Current contraceptive issues

Depomedroxyprogesterone

There has been a drive to limit the use of depo in younger women and to limit the duration of use to 2 years, following a better understanding of the effects on the bone mineral density.

Depomedroxyprogesterone and bone mineral density (BMD)
J Fam Plann Reprod Health Care **2002; 28(1): 12–15**

This study of 48 women, each with over 2 years of DMPA use for contraception, found that BMD of the femoral neck (FN) and the lumbar spine (LS) showed significant reduction. Mean Z score: LS -0.84 (95% CI 1.17 to -0.52); FN 0.32 (95% CI 0.62 to -0.2).

Evra patch (norelgestromin and ethinyloestradiol)

This was licensed in the UK in 2003. It is worn for 3 weeks out of a 4-week cycle and the patch needs to be changed weekly.

New product review (Sept 2003) Norelgestromin/ethinyloestradiol transdermal contraceptive patch (EVRA)
J Fam Plann Reprod Health Care **2004; 30(1): 43–5**

The overall Pearl Index was 1.24 (95% CI 0.19–2.33), similar to triphasic contraceptive pills. Self-reported compliance was 10% better with the patch (88.2%) compared with the pill (77.7%). This is an additional choice for women wanting combined hormonal contraception.

Yasmin

This is a combined contraceptive with anti-mineralocorticoid activity, which has a role to play in treating hirsute polycystic ovary patients. There is no substantiated evidence that any initial weight loss is maintained (a claim withdrawn by the marketing company).

Immunocontraception

A novel approach that is receiving a considerable degree of attention. Sperm have unique proteins, and targeting antibodies to these gamete-specific antigens could be successful. Vaccines targeting the hCG molecule are currently undergoing phase I and phase II trials in humans.

Folic acid supplemented contraception
This is being given consideration as there are still some preventable foetal abnormalities occurring. It would help, for example, in women who stop the pill to conceive but forget to take folic acid.

Emergency contraception

A MORI survey revealed that 43% of 15- to 24-year-olds reported that they had had casual sex at some time in the past 10 years, and that 40% of these had failed to use a condom. Around 12% of patients who require emergency contraception are under 16 years of age. Emergency contraception is available free on prescription from GPs, family planning clinics, youth clinics, walk-in centres, genito-urinary clinics, and some Accident and Emergency departments and pharmacists.

In 1983, the Attorney General ruled that emergency contraception is not a form of abortion as there is no pregnancy to terminate. This was further supported in 2002.

Awareness of emergency contraception
J Fam Plann Reprod Health Care **2005; 32(2): 113–14**

In this study of 78 women who attended for termination, 60% felt that emergency contraception was easily available, but only 37% of them had ever used it. It concluded that there are many reasons why emergency contraception is underused.

Levonelle is now the first-line treatment, although PC4 is still available and has been shown to be effective with a stat dose of 1.5 mg (this dose became available as a single tablet in November 2005). Levonelle has been available from pharmacists since January 2001 following pilot studies that showed a high demand, that patients were using the drug appropriately and that it was safe. The demand through pharmacists is increasing (especially following the new pharmacy contract), and the Office for National Statistics has published data showing that demand through pharmacists has increased from 27% (2003/04) to 50% (2004/05), while that through GPs has fallen from 41% to 33%.

If a patient weighs over 70 kg, the Oxford Family Planning Association study has confirmed a higher failure rate of progesterone-only pills. Advice for levonelle is that patients take one 1.5 mg tablet as soon as possible after unprotected sexual intercourse and repeat the dose after 12 hours (a 100% increase in the dose). This also follows for women on enzyme-inducing drugs, but is not evidence based. Women should be warned of the greater risk of ectopic pregnancy following emergency contraception.

Community pharmacy supply of emergency hormonal contraception (EHC): a structured literature review of international evidence
Hum Reprod **2005; Sept 2**

This systematic review (January 1990 to January 2005) included 24 peer-reviewed papers: one randomised controlled trial and 23 qualitative or observational studies.

The pharmacy supply of EHC enables most women to receive it within 24 hours of unprotected intercourse, which is a feature rated highly by women. The randomised controlled trial showed that it did not reduce the use of other contraceptive methods, neither did it lead to an increase in risky sexual behaviour and infection. One study found that pharmacy supply has led to a reduction in women's Accident and Emergency attendance. (These data were further supported by an article; the *BMJ* **2005; 331: 271–3**.)

Advance supply of emergency contraception: a randomized trial in adolescent mothers
J Pediatr Adolesc Gynecol **2005; 18(5): 347–54**

This study looked at 160 mothers aged 13–20 years, interviewing them at 6 and then 12 months post partum. They found that if they had EHC issued 'just in case', they were much more likely to use EHC, that it did not affect use of condoms or other methods of contraception but they were more likely to have unprotected sex. (A further study has shown that issuing EHC in this way does not reduce abortion rates; *Contraception* **2004; 69: 361–6**.)

Other options for emergency contraception
Don't forget that an IUD can be used up to 5 days after unprotected intercourse (i.e. up to day 19 of a regular 28-day cycle). Medicolegally, this is not procuring an abortion (it has been tested in the courts).

Improving teenagers' knowledge of contraception: cluster RCT of teacher-led intervention
BMJ **2002; 324: 1179–83**

This study found that teachers giving a single lesson on emergency contraception to year 10 pupils improved the number of boys and girls who knew the correct time limits for both types of emergency contraception. It did not change sexual activity or use of emergency contraception.

Teenage pregnancy

The age of consent (from a legal perspective) to any form of sexual activity is 16 for both men and women. There is a series of laws to help protect children aged 13 to 16 years from abuse, and the maximum sentence for the rape of a child under 13 years is life imprisonment. There is no defence of mistaken belief about age as there is in 13- to 15-year-olds.

Teenage sexual health, pregnancy and termination are always topical, and are currently more so following the publication of advice that all health professionals will be legally obliged to report all sexual activity in adolescents under 16 years of age to the police. This is in line with the new national child protection guidelines *Working Together to Safeguard Children*. This reporting will be irrespective of whether you feel there is an issue of abuse, and it is being contested – the fear being that mandatory reporting will be too blunt an instrument and will stop teenagers seeking sexual health advice, contraception and antenatal care.

Teenage Pregnancy Unit statistics have found the following.

- In England there are 39,600 conceptions per year to teenagers.
- The teenage (under-18) conception rate is 42–48 per 1,000 conceptions per year and almost half lead to termination.
- Nationally, the rate is starting to fall (London remained stable from 1998 to 2003), but we still have the highest teenage pregnancy rate in Western Europe.
- In England, a total of 174,000 terminations are performed each year and 12.4% of these are to women under 18 years, following either a previous birth (5%) or previous termination (7.4%).
- One in every ten babies in the UK is born to a teenage mother.

It is well recognised that teenage pregnancies:

- are seen at higher rates in deprived areas
- mean that teenage mothers are less likely to finish their education or find a job
- mean teenage mothers are more likely to bring their children up in poverty
- generally lead to poorer antenatal health and low birth-weight babies
- when resulting in a birth, mean the infants have twice the mortality rate seen in the population.

Health of the Nation 1990

This initiative increased priorities for under-16s and aimed to halve the rate of teenage pregnancies by 2000. This goal was not met for a number of reasons, including the fact that GPs have little influence on risk-taking behaviour.

Modernising Health and Social Services 2000/01 to 2002/03

This highlights the tackling of teenage pregnancies in light of the *Health of the Nation* findings, especially preventing conception and supporting teenage parents.

National Teenage Pregnancy Strategy

www.dfes.gov.uk/teenagepregnancy/dsp
This strategy is set out in the *Social Exclusion Unit Report on Teenage Pregnancy Issues* and was launched in 1999 with the following aims:

- to halve under-18 conception rates in England by 2010
- to increase the participation of teenage mothers in education, training or work by 60% by 2010, to reduce the risk of long-term social exclusion.

Issues relating to teenage pregnancies

1 *Provision of health and sex education*: teenagers are often unaware of how to obtain contraceptive advice and believe they have to be over 16 years of age to obtain treatment. However, since the Gillick ruling of October 1985 (the Fraser guidelines), this is no longer the case. Teenagers are often willing to run the risk of sexually transmitted infections and pregnancy because they think their parents will find out if they see their GP (confidentiality is needed at all levels).

2 *Contraceptive services need to be accessible*: this includes GPs/family planning services/ school nurses/youth clinics, etc.

3 *Role of schools*: this includes sex education/behavioural interventions, as well as the need to develop communication skills and sustain the truth that virginity still prevails among the majority (apparently).

Teenagers' use of sexual health services: perceived need, knowledge and ability to access
J Fam Plann Reprod Health Care 2004; 30(4): 217–24

In this study, 5,747 15- and 16-year-olds were questioned about their use of sexual health services. The key points were that effective school sex education was associated with an increased uptake of services. Sexual experience, proximity to clinics, parental influences, knowledge and confidence were all associated with service use. Also that boys' uptake of services may be improved through better knowledge, greater confidence and peer-group discussion.

Positive experiences of teenage motherhood: a qualitative study
Br J Gen Pract 2004; 54: 813–18

This was a small study of nine teenage mothers. They had recognised that they were still young enough to further their education and were realistic about their futures, making plans for their careers. A nice twist, showing that it doesn't have to be all doom and gloom.

Breast cancer

This accounted for 27% of all female cancers in 1995. It is the most common female cancer and it is the cause of 18% of all female deaths.

Around 5% of all breast cancers are linked to specific single gene defects, 80% of which are due to BRCA 1 or 2.

Breast screening

The NHS breast screening programme was introduced in England and Wales in 1988 on the recommendation of the Forrest Committee. In 2002, the Department of Health report showed that screening women aged 55–64 years of age had increased from 75.6% in 2001 to 76.2% in 2002. In one year, 1.3 million women were screened and

8,345 cancers were diagnosed using mammography. Mammography is currently the best tool for screening for breast cancer and it is offered to all women aged 50–70 years of age every 3 years (women over 70 years may request ongoing 3-yearly screening).

Scientists are developing salivary tests that measure genetic markers of cancer. Although these will not replace mammography for many years, the tests so far predict breast (and oral) cancers with 95% accuracy.

The Leningrad and Shanghai studies are large, randomised controlled trials that have both failed to demonstrate a reduction in mortality from breast cancer or increased detection by teaching self-examination.

Mammography has been shown in a Swedish randomised controlled trial to reduce mortality by up to 40%, the benefit being greatest in those aged 50–70 years. Compared with symptomatic breast cancers, screen-detected cancers are smaller and more likely to be non-invasive. If they are invasive, they are more likely to be better differentiated and node-negative.

Efficacy of breast cancer screening in the community according to risk level
J Natl Canc Instit 2005; 97: 1035–43

This was a community-based, matched, case-controlled study in the USA of 1,351 case subjects. It found that there was no appreciable association between breast cancer mortality and screening history (odds ratio 0.92; 95% CI 0.76–1.13) in the community setting.

It has been calculated that for every 2 million women screened, one extra cancer after 10 years may be caused by the radiation delivered to the breast from mammography.

No increase in anxiety has been found in women invited to attend for screening unless there is a need for recall.

HRT reduces the sensitivity of mammography (from 77% to 65%) and is associated with more false positives.

Effect of NHS Breast Screening Programme on mortality from breast cancer in England and Wales, 1990–98: comparison of observed with predicted mortality
BMJ 2000; 321: 665–9

This study showed that in women aged 40–79 years, there has been a 21% fall in mortality since 1991, 6% due to screening and 15% to treatment. The covering editorial (*BMJ* 2000; 321: 647–8) discusses factors other than mortality when determining success of a screening programme.

Model outcome of screening mammography: information to support informed choices
BMJ 2005; 330: 936–8

Risk and benefit should be set out in a more straightforward way for patients using decision-making models. This paper presents age-specific estimates of benefits and harms of screening mammography.

- For every 1,000 women screened over 10 years, 167–251 (depending on age) receive an abnormal result and are recalled.

- About 56–64 of these have at least one biopsy.

- 9–26 have an invasive cancer detected by screening.

- About 0.5, two, three and two fewer deaths from breast cancer occur every 10 years per 1,000 women aged 40, 50, 60 and 70 years respectively who choose to be screened compared with those who don't.

Cervical cancer

www.cancerresearchuk.org

- The incidence of cervical cancer in the UK is 9.6 per 100,000.

- The mortality rate is 5 per 100,000.

- The incidence of disease peaks at 30–35 and 70–75 years of age.

- Around 95% of cervical cancers are squamous cell and 5% are adenocarcinomas.

- The most important risk factor is human papillomavirus (HPV). At least 50% of sexually active people will get HPV (type 16, 18, 31, 33 or 35). Smoking and the age at first intercourse are also important factors.

Cervical screening

- This may prevent cervical cancer completely.

- Around 80% of women aged 25–64 years have been screened (3.8 million women).

- Cervical screening prevents around 5,000 deaths per year in the UK. The incidence of cervical cancer fell by 42% between 1988 and 1996 (in England and Wales) as a direct consequence of the cervical screening programme.

Protocol for cervical screening

Age group	Frequency
25	First invitation
25–49	3-yearly invitation
50–64	5-yearly invitation
Over 65	Only if the last three tests include an abnormal result

Prevalence of high-grade CIN following mild dyskaryotic smears in different age groups
Cytopathology 2005; 16(6): 277–80

The British Society of Colposcopy and Cervical Pathology recommend colposcopy after one mildly dyskaryotic smear. This study looked at 510 women from April 2000 to March 2003. The overall prevalence of CIN II and III was 28.7%, and this was similar in all age groups. The concern here is that a significant number of women under 25 years of age (age of first screening) may have a high-grade CIN for over 5 years before they become eligible for screening.

Liquid-based cytology
In conventional smear taking a wooden spatula or brush is used to transfer cells on to a slide. However, up to 80% of cervical cells are not transferred from the spatula or brush to the slide. In 2003, it was announced that liquid-based cytology (LBC) would become the test of choice in the UK.

- LBC reduces inadequate smears from 9% to 2%.

- LBC is currently a more expensive option, but a cost saving would be made by a reduced need for repeats.

- The sample brush is sent to the laboratory in a vial of fluid. The fluid is then spun down and the cells are filtered out under pressure on to a slide, which is then analysed.

Human papillomavirus

The Health Technology Assessment Report concluded that the clearest role for HPV testing was in the management of women with borderline or mild dyskaryotic smears, to enable those testing positive for a high-risk group to be referred for colposcopy.

A negative HPV test virtually rules out any abnormality being present. The methods used at present are still being improved, as there are too many false positives.

Human papillomavirus vaccine
Around 95% of all cervical cancer is attributed to HPV, and development of a vaccine that may prevent this is one of the most exciting developments in modern medicine.

Gardasil (the quadrivalent HPV 6, 11, 16 and 18 recombinant vaccine) has been found to prevent 100% of cases of high-grade pre-cancerous lesions, as well as non-invasive cancers (CIN II and III or AIS) associated with HPV 16 and 18. This was seen after a 2-year follow-up of a three-dose regime.

The need for booster vaccines, changes to the cervical screening programme, the therapeutic role of vaccines and cost-effectiveness (as well as whether men should be included in the vaccination programme) are all areas that will need clarification.

Human papillomavirus (HPV) vaccines: prospects for eradicating cervical cancer
J Fam Plann Reprod Health Care 2004; 30(40): 213–15

This editorial gives an interesting overview of prophylactic vaccines and their development, as well as insight into their therapeutic use. Margaret Stanley (professor of epithelial biology) holds the view that these vaccines will be licensed within the next 5 years.

Ovarian cancer

- Ovarian cancer is the fourth most common female cancer in the UK.

- The incidence in the UK is 20 per 100,000 (and it appears to be increasing).

- Each year there are 6,900 new cases.

- Women with BRCA 1 gene have a 50% lifetime risk, and those with BRCA 2 have a 30% lifetime risk (the same risk as if two first-degree relatives have ovarian cancer).

Ovarian screening

There is no proven role for screening, but methods would include Ca125 and transvaginal ultrasound scanning. In some areas, women with one or more first-degree relatives with ovarian cancer may be offered a yearly Ca125 and ultrasound scan. They should be made aware of the limitations of these methods, and the lack of evidence for this approach. Trials looking at the success of screening for ovarian cancer have not been encouraging.

The Medical Research Council has launched a 10-year trial (UK Collaborative Trial of Ovarian Cancer Screening) of 200,000 postmenopausal women, looking at transvaginal ultrasound scan versus Ca125 on a yearly basis to try to establish the effectiveness of each method in terms of their impact on mortality, morbidity and cost.

Yale University has isolated 35 proteins which are significantly higher in women with ovarian cancer, and is currently validating the use of four (leptin, prolactin, osteopontin and insulin-like growth factor-2).

Antenatal care

In October 2003, NICE published its guidance on antenatal care, *Routine care for healthy pregnant women*, and the NSF for Children, Young People and Maternity Services was published in 2004. This looks at all areas from preconception, pre-birth and birth to postnatal community care.

Down's syndrome screening

Down's syndrome is the most common chromosomal abnormality at birth. The incidence is related to maternal age, and the Down's syndrome screening programme is part of antenatal modernisation.

By 2007, NICE indicates that pregnant women should be offered the following tests (which would provide detection rates above 75%).

- From 11 to 14 weeks:
  - the combined test (nuchal translucency (NT), hCG and PAPP-A).

- From 14 to 20 weeks:
  - the quadruple test (hCG, AFP, uE3, inhibin A).

- From 11 to 14 weeks and 14 to 20 weeks:
  - the integrated test (NT, PAPP-A + hCG, AFP, uE3, inhibin A)
  - the serum integrated test (PAPP-A + hCG, AFP, uE3, inhibin A).

Retrospective audit of different antenatal screening policies for Down's syndrome in eight district general hospitals in one health region
BMJ 2002; 325: 15–17

These audit results showed that serum screening for Down's syndrome did not improve detection or reduce the number of cases needing amniocentesis. Thus serum tests and nuchal translucency screening may be less advantageous than previously thought.

Since March 2001 all NHS regions should have had a Down's syndrome co-ordinator in post, and by 2004 each hospital should have a local co-ordinator to develop services and offer support to GPs, midwives and pregnant women.

HIV testing

- If an HIV-infected woman is unaware of her infection status, her baby has around a one in four chance of being infected.

- Around 300 babies each year are born with HIV (mainly in London).

- Up to 80% of these cases could be prevented by the use of antivirals (antenatally, during delivery and for the infant), lower-segment Caesarean section and avoiding breastfeeding.

Women are now being offered HIV screening at booking to reduce the risk of transmission (national targets were adopted in 1999). Although screening is offered, there is not always the necessary counselling available to fully explain the implications of not having the test or a positive test. Previously there was a need for documented written consent, but HIV testing antenatally is now becoming a more acceptable routine test given the scope of available treatment for the neonate and the mother.

Social and ethical inequalities in the offer and uptake of prenatal screening and diagnosis in the UK: a systematic review
Public Health 2004; 118(3): 177–89

This systematic review identified 20 relevant papers. None found any significant social inequalities in testing, although some suggested that women of South Asian origin might be up to 70% less likely to receive prenatal testing for haemoglobin disorders and Down's syndrome than white women. They concluded that there may be some evidence of ethnic inequalities to prenatal testing, but there is little understanding behind why.

Pre-eclampsia

This condition complicates around 10% of pregnancies. There are many theories on the reasons for development of pre-eclampsia: genetics (maternal, paternal and foetal), raised homocysteine levels in initially normotensive women and Leiden factor V gene are all being given consideration in current journals. US research has shown that there may be a window in the first trimester for detection of pre-eclampsia using sex hormone-binding globulin as a marker. This is not currently used.

Risk factors for pre-eclampsia at antenatal booking: systematic review of controlled trials
BMJ 2005; 330: 565–7

The authors looked at trials published from 1966 to 2002 and found an increased risk in the following cohorts:

- a previous history of pre-eclampsia (relative risk 7.19, 95% CI 5.85–8.83)
- the presence of antiphospholipid antibodies (relative risk 9.72, 95% CI 4.34–21.75)
- pre-existing diabetes (relative risk 3.56, 95% CI 2.54–4.99)
- twin pregnancies (relative risk 2.93, 95% CI 2.04–4.21)
- nulliparity (relative risk 2.91, 95% CI 1.28–6.61).

Family history, raised blood pressure (>80 mmHg diastolic) at booking, maternal age over 40 years, raised BMI before pregnancy and multiparous women were also shown to increase the risk.

World Health Organization systematic review of screening tests for pre-eclampsia
Obstet Gynecol 2004; 104 (6): 1367–91
This study looked for evidence for the usefulness of clinical, biophysical and biochemical tests in the prediction of pre-eclampsia (in data from 1966 to February 2003). It concluded that as of 2004, there is no useful screening test to predict the development of pre-eclampsia.

The pre-eclampsia community guideline (PRECOG): how to screen for and detect onset of pre-eclampsia in the community
BMJ 2005; 330: 576–80

This is a simple, comprehensive guideline giving a structured approach to the risk assessments we make for our antenatal patients. It was developed because 46% of maternal deaths and 65% of foetal deaths due to pre-eclampsia could have had a different outcome if they had been managed differently. It looks at assessment in early pregnancy, referral criteria to specialist units and community monitoring. Important signs and symptoms to identify are: new hypertension, new proteinuria, headaches and/or visual disturbance, epigastric pain and/or vomiting, reduced foetal movements and babies that are small for their gestational age. The only weakness identified is the lack of evidence to support recommendations of more frequent assessment. Although criteria for screening have not been met, this is not a concern that will limit the implementation of this commonsense, workable guide.

There is the theoretical belief that anti-platelets may have a role in prophylaxis, but there is a lot of conflicting evidence. The CLASP trial and subsequent meta-analyses showed no benefit. Use of aspirin in women at high risk of early-onset pre-eclampsia may be beneficial.

Low-dose aspirin in pregnancy and early childhood development: follow-up of the collaborative low-dose aspirin study in pregnancy. CLASP Collaborative group
Br J Obstet Gynaecol **1995; 102 (11): 861–8**

This was the 12- and 18-month follow-up of children born to women who had been at high risk of complications from pre-eclampsia. The findings were reassuring about the safety of aspirin, but it showed no clear evidence of benefit.

Postnatal depression

Drug Ther Bull **2000; 38(5): 33–7**

- One in 10 women become depressed after childbirth (70,000 women/year).

- Around 50% are still having problems 6 months postnatally.

- This is different from 'baby blues', which is common around days 3–5 (up to day 10), does not require treatment and it is less severe than puerperal psychosis.

- Postnatal depression tends to start around 4–6 weeks after delivery.

- It is important to diagnose and treat early to minimise problems with bonding within the family.

Edinburgh Postnatal Depression Scale
Br J Psych **1987; 150: 782–876**

This scale was developed in primary care to improve detection through screening. It is used at 6–8 weeks postnatally and is scored by a health professional (GP, health visitor or midwife).

1 I have been able to laugh and see the funny side of things.
   As much as I always could   0
   Not quite so much now   1
   Definitely not so much now   2
   Not at all   3

2 I have looked forward with enjoyment to things.

As much as I ever did 0

Rather less than I used to 1

Definitely less than I used to 2

Hardly at all 3

3 I have blamed myself unnecessarily when thing went wrong.

Yes, most of the time 3

Yes some of the time 2

Not very often 1

No, never 0

4 I have been anxious or worried for no good reason.

No not at all 0

Hardly ever 1

Yes sometimes 2

Yes very often 3

5 I have felt scared or panicky for no good reason.

Yes quite a lot 3

Yes sometimes 2

No not much 1

No not at all 0

6 Things have been getting on top of me.

Yes most of the time I haven't been able to cope at all 3

Yes sometimes I haven't been coping as well as usual 2

No most of the time I have coped quite well 1

No I have been coping as well as ever 0

7 I have been so unhappy that I have had difficulty sleeping.

Yes most of the time 3

Yes sometimes 2

Not very often 1

No not at all 0

8 I have felt sad or miserable.

Yes most of the time 3

Yes quite often 2

Not very often 1

No not at all 0

9 I have been so unhappy that I have been crying.

Yes most of the time 3

Yes quite often 2

Only occasionally 1

No never 0

10 The thought of harming myself has occurred to me.

Yes quite often 3

Sometimes 2

Hardly ever 1

Never 0

If the calculated total score is >13 then there is a 92.3% chance that the woman is suffering from a depressive illness. The score should not override clinical judgement.

Treatment of postnatal depression

Treatment of proven benefit includes cognitive behavioural therapy and counselling by a health visitor. SSRIs and tricyclic antidepressants appear to be safe in breast-feeding women.

Psychosocial and psychological interventions for prevention of postnatal depression: systematic review
BMJ 2005; 331: 15–18

This study took into account results of several different trials (7,697 women) and found that diverse psychosocial or psychological interventions do not significantly reduce the number of women who develop postnatal depression. The most promising intervention was the provision of individual intensive, professionally-based, post-partum care (relative risk 0.76, 95% CI 0.59–1.0).

Confidential Inquiry into Maternal Deaths, 1997–1999
This found a small reduction in deaths from obstetric causes. However, there was an increase in deaths in women who had concurrent medical or psychological problems. The leading cause of death was from suicide during the postnatal period.

Men's health

Several studies have shown that men seek help for a given illness later than women. Although they do care about health issues, they find it more difficult to express their fears.

Prostate cancer

www.doh.gov.uk/cancer/prostate.htm

- Prostate cancer is the second most common cause of cancer-related deaths in men in the UK. Around 9,500 men die from the disease each year.
- Around 20,000 new cases are diagnosed each year.
- Around 25% of men with a prostate-specific antigen (PSA) level of 4–10 ng/ml will be found to have cancer.
- Around 20% of men with prostate cancer do not have a raised PSA.
- Around 60% of cases have metastatic disease at the time of diagnosis.

PSA is the current tumour marker being used when investigating for prostate cancer. Its use for a population-based screening programme is being evaluated in a prospective randomised trial, the outcome of which will be known in around five years.

Although there is no screening programme, any man can have a PSA test if he requests one. Hence screening may creep in, although it doesn't satisfy the criteria for a screening programme. Evidence is lacking that screening for prostate cancer would be beneficial.

Arguments against screening with PSA include the following.

- There is a lack of consensus on treatment for early disease and a risk of harm with diagnostic biopsy.

- Despite the widespread use of PSA testing there is lack of evidence that it reduces mortality.

- Up to 20% of prostate cancers will not raise the PSA.

- Only a minority of cancers spread to shorten life expectancy.

- The PSA is unable to distinguish between indolent and aggressive tumours.

- PSA is not tumour specific and can also be raised in prostatitis, benign prostatic hypertrophy, urinary retention, instrumentation and ejaculation.

- There is no specific cut-off below which the risk of prostate cancer is zero.

Screening decreases prostate cancer mortality: 11-year follow-up of the 1988 Quebec prospective randomised controlled trial
Prostate **2004; 59(3): 311–18**

Two studies have now found that yearly screening reduces mortality by as much as 8%. This particular study looked at 46,486 men aged 45–80 years in Quebec and found that 74 deaths due to prostate cancer occurred in the unscreened group compared to 10 deaths in the screened group (mean follow-up of 7.93 years). The statistics used were a Cox proportional hazards model of the age at death from prostate cancer, which showed a 62% reduction ($p < 0.002$) in screened men.

Individualised screening interval for prostate cancer based on PSA level: results of a prospective, randomised population-based study
Arch Intern Med **2005; 165(16): 1857–61**

The study included 5,855 men aged 50 to 66 years who had accepted the invitation to take part in the study. Men with a PSA >3.0 ng/ml were offered a biopsy. After a mean follow-up of 7.6 years, 539 cases (9.2%) of cancer were detected. If the PSA was found to be less than 1 ng/ml, then not a single case developed prostate cancer within 3 years. They concluded that the resting interval should be individualised, based on PSA level at the time of testing.

Prostate cancer vaccine

Prostate-specific membrane antigen (PSMA) has been a target for vaccines, as has radioactively labelled monoclonal antibodies against PSMA. Although certain vaccines are in the clinical trial phase, as yet there are no conclusive results on efficacy.

Benign prostatic hypertrophy

- Around 3.3 million men in the UK have benign prostatic hypertrophy (BPH).

- The prime concern in management, besides symptom control, is to ensure that those men with outflow obstruction do not go on to develop renal failure.

The International Prostate Symptom Score (IPSS) is one way of assessing symptoms over time with treatment, and the BPH Impact Index is a way of assessing how troublesome symptoms are.

Management

1 *Alpha-blockers* (e.g. prazosin, indoramin). These relax the smooth muscle of the prostate. In randomised controlled trials they have proved more effective than placebo. They usually produce an improvement within 2–3 weeks. If there is no improvement within 3–4 months, an alternative should be tried.

2 *5-alpha-reductase inhibitors* (e.g. finasteride). These inhibit 5-alpha-reductase, which converts testosterone to dihydroxytestosterone (DHT), and is known to influence prostate growth. Randomised controlled trials have confirmed that they are more effective than placebo. They cause hyperplasia to regress over 3–6 months (allow 12 months for maximum effect), so are especially suitable if the prostate is enlarged. They may reduce the PSA by up to 50%.

Impact of baseline symptom severity on future risk of benign prostatic hyperplasia-related outcomes and long-term response to finasteride. The PLESS study group
Urology **2000; 56(4): 610–16**

The Proscar long-term efficacy and safety study has published several outcome studies. A total of 3,040 men with BPH were treated for 4 years with either finasteride or placebo. Finasteride reduced the risk of surgery and acute urinary retention in all groups ($p < 0.001$).

3 *Plant extracts.*
- Saw palmetto (*Serona repens*) (Permixon). This is an extract from a cactus-like plant. It has had some success (although the trial did not use a placebo arm) and is thought to work in a similar way to finasteride.
- β-sitosterol. Trials have shown that this is more effective than placebo in the short term. The side effects include gastrointestinal symptoms and impotence.
- Rye grass pollen extract. It has been suggested that this is beneficial, but trials as yet are inconclusive.

4 *Botulinum A toxin.* When this is injected into the prostate it has been shown to improve symptoms of BPH.

Erectile dysfunction

www.bhf.org.uk/factfiles

- Around 50% of men aged 40–70 years experience some degree of erectile dysfunction (ED).
- ED is frequently a manifestation of underlying vascular disease, and men should be screened for risk factors and signs of vascular disease as part of the assessment.
- The incidence is doubled in men with hypertension, tripled in those with diabetes and quadrupled in men with coronary heart disease.
- Cigarette smoking increases the prevalence of all of the above twofold.

If there is a normal libido and secondary sexual characteristics, it is unusual to find a low testosterone level. If sex hormone-binding globulin (SHBG) and testosterone levels are requested, a ratio can then be determined (i.e. the availability of testosterone), which may help management.

Treatment

Involve the partner as well as the patient where possible. Patients who received an NHS prescription before 14 September 1998 can continue to receive erectile dysfunction treatment (not just the first method they were prescribed) on the NHS (the script should be endorsed 'SLS'). Otherwise, treatment is only available on the NHS for patients with certain medical problems, e.g. prostate cancer, diabetes, spinal cord injury, Parkinson's disease, multiple sclerosis (there are 12 in total). Private scripts can be written for those not eligible for NHS treatment.

Phosphodiesterase type 5 (PDE) inhibitors (sildenafil, tadalafil and vardenafil)
These are selective inhibitors of phosphodiesterase type 5, and are currently the favoured option, but are contra-indicated in patients taking nitrates. The best responders are those with psychogenic causes, and they are mainly effective in arousal because they prolong the production of nitric oxide (a vasodilator). The response seen may be less marked after around 2 years of use. There is an understanding that if the treatment is used regularly the response is better than if it is used infrequently.

An open-label, multicentre, randomised cross-over study comparing sildenafil citrate and tadalafil for treating erectile dysfunction in men naive to phosphodiesterase 5 inhibitor therapy
Br J Urol 2005; 96(9): 1323–32

Following a 4-week baseline assessment, 367 men with ED (average age of 54 years) were randomised to receive sildenafil for 12 weeks followed by tadalafil for 12 weeks, or vice versa. Both treatments were seen to be effective. After treatment, 29% of men chose sildenafil and 71% chose tadalafil for an 8-week extension. Tadalafil is known to have a 24-hour duration of action and to work within 30 minutes, so although it is more expensive, you usually get 'more bang for your buck'.

Apomorphine (Uprima) (dopamine receptor agonist)
This drug has been licensed for ED. Currently there are no prescribing restrictions. There is a 1 in 500 risk of syncope due to vasovagal response, so care is needed with the first dose and when increasing from 2 to 3 mg.

Intra-cavernosal prostaglandin E₁ (alprostadil)
Around 80% of men have a satisfactory erection with this method, but they need to be taught how to self-inject.

Intra-urethral prostaglandin E₁
The Muse system of pellets is used. Around 30% of men report some discomfort after use, which can cause discontinuation of treatment. One randomised controlled trial showed a satisfactory effect in 40% of men.

Yohimbine (alpha-blocker)
This drug is not yet licensed. It has been found to be effective in some placebo controlled trials, but its effectiveness is probably inadequate for treatment of most ED.

National Strategy for Sexual Health and HIV (2001)

www.doh.gov.uk
www.sxhealth.co.uk

In July 2001, a consultation document was published that outlined the Government's proposed strategy for sexual health and HIV. The main aim of the strategy is to prevent sexual causes of premature deaths and ill health, as well as to ensure that services are available for those patients who need them.

Local networks of providers will be based on three service levels.

Level 1: to be provided by GPs

- Sexual history and risk assessment.

- Contraceptive information and services.

- Pregnancy testing and referral.

- Cervical cytology screening and referral.

- Sexually transmitted disease (STD) testing for women.

- Assessment and referral for men.

- HIV testing and counselling.

- Hepatitis B immunisation.

Level 2: intermediate care to be provided by primary care teams with a special interest (e.g. an enhanced service), genito-urinary medicine or family planning clinics

- IUD and contraceptive implants.
- Testing and treatment of STDs.
- Invasive STD testing for men.
- Partner notification and contact tracing.
- Vasectomy.

Level 3: specialist clinical teams across more than one primary care group

- Outreach contraceptive services.
- Outreach STD prevention.
- Specialised infection management, including contact tracing.
- Specialised HIV treatment and care.

A large proportion of GPs already provide Level 1 services (the exception being HIV testing). GPs could take on extra work now as part of an enhanced service within the new contract.

A Sexual Health Strategy for England
BMJ 2001; 323: 243–4

This article gives an overview of some of the issues. The £47.5 million to be invested between 2002 and 2004 was thought to be insufficient at the time. If the target for reducing HIV and gonorrhoea by 25% by 2007 is met, it could save the Government £450 million. It was felt that the document was more concerned with disease prevention rather than health promotion. Abuse and assault services were not highlighted.

Sexual health care training needs of general practitioner trainers: a regional survey
J Fam Plann Reprod Health Care 2005; 31(3): 213–18

Following the aims of the sexual health strategy to improve access to sexual health care primarily in general practice, this study surveyed 374 GPs (295 of these questionnaires were returned, 79%). The main drawback with regard to implementation (from GPs at ground level) was the training needed – 82% felt considerably more training was needed to support the strategy.

Chlamydia

- Reported rates of chlamydia are 1,339 in 100,000 in 16 to 19-year-olds, rising steadily (9%) from 2002 to 2003.

- Around 70% of women and 50% of men are asymptomatic. There may be non-specific symptoms.

- The cost to the NHS is £100 million per year to treat chlamydia and its complications.

- It is the most common curable sexually transmitted disease in Europe.

- It can cause ectopic pregnancy, pelvic inflammatory disease (in 10–30% of cases), infertility and perihepatitis (Fitz-Hugh–Curtis Syndrome), and there can be neo-natal transmission.

High-risk groups are 16 to 25-year-olds and women undergoing a termination of pregnancy. Behavioural risk factors include teenagers leaving school at a young age, women with multiple partners, being single and people from ethnic minorities.

Evaluation of nucleic acid amplification tests (NAATs) in the absence of a perfect gold standard test: a review of the statistical and epidemiological issues
Epidemiology 2005; 16(5): 604–12

This is an interesting insight into the limitations of NAATs, polymerase chain reaction, ligase chain reaction and transcription-mediated amplification tests in diagnostic testing for sexually transmitted diseases. It found that NAATs (currently used as the test of choice in the UK) had a sensitivity of around 97.6% and a specificity of 95.3%.

Screening for chlamydia

In 1996, the Chief Medical Officer's Advisory Group called for a national screening programme and, following pilot studies, the Chlamydia Screening Programme was outlined in the National Strategy for Sexual Health and HIV. The aim is to implement this for men and women under 25 years of age by 2008.

Chief Medical Officer's Report
BMJ 1998; 316: 351

This recommended opportunistic screening of the following:

- sexually active women under 25 years of age

- older women with a new partner or two or more partners in the last year.

It also recommended including the following groups on clinical grounds:

- patients attending genito-urinary medicine clinics

- women undergoing termination of pregnancy

- high-risk groups and prior to instrumentation (including IUCDs).

It is important not to confuse opportunistic screening of asymptomatic men and women with the need for a full complement of swabs and bloods tests in high-risk individuals, where it is important to consider all sexually transmitted infections.

National Chlamydia Screening Programme
www.doh.gov.uk

This was launched in 2003, with the following aims:

- controlling chlamydia through early detection and treatment of asymptomatic infection
- reducing onward transmission
- preventing the consequences of untreated infection.

Initially, ten opportunistic screening programmes were implemented in 2002, with a further 16 programmes being announced in 2004 (currently covering 25% of primary care trusts in England). Over 78,000 people have been screened so far (a threefold increase was seen from 2003 to 2004), with 8,000 positive results. By 2008, the programme is intended to be national.

In men, a first-pass urine has 75–100% sensitivity and in women a self-taken vulvo-vaginal swab has over 80% sensitivity with 99% specificity (urine in women has been shown to be less sensitive). Endocervical swabs at the time of a cervical smear may also be used.

The following criteria have to be fulfilled to achieve the aims of screening:

- include all sexually active men and women
- include people under 25 years of age
- include only asymptomatic people (if symptomatic then complete investigation is needed)
- contacts of positive patients need to be traced.

Although the screening is initiated in primary care (general practice, antenatal clinics, family planning, colposcopy clinics, etc.), the chlamydia screening office then co-ordinates the result notification, treatment if needed (azithromycin 1 g stat is first-line treatment, taking 1 week to work) and contact tracing.

The person undergoing the test has the option of receiving the results by phone (text messaging is offered in some regions) or in person.

Further pilots are in place, with Boots the Chemist looking at their role in offering screening.

Screening implications for general practitioners
1 Extra time is needed by clinical staff:
  – for taking samples from at-risk patients or explaining how to do a self-test
  – for training of practice staff

– for taking a sexual history from all patients under 25 years
– for pre-test counselling
– for counselling patients who test positive. Although the office will co-ordinate things it is inevitable that there will be some fall out
– for partner notification and treatment
– to ensure compliance and follow-up to treatment.

2 Extra resources are needed:
   – for staff training
   – for laboratory tests.

3 Issues:
   – compliance requires sexual abstinence for 1 week
   – contact tracing (6-month history from patients)
   – consider a test of cure
   – genito-urinary referral confidentiality issue, insurance forms, etc.

Postal screening
Coverage and uptake of systematic postal screening for genital *Chlamydia trachomatis* and prevalence of infection in the UK general population: cross-sectional survey
BMJ **2005; 330: 940–2**

This cross-sectional survey invited 19,773 men and women aged 16–39 years of age to participate in screening, with 73% coverage (uptake in 16- to 24-year-olds was 31.5%). The overall prevalence of chlamydia was 2.8%. It concluded that postal screening was feasible, but coverage was incomplete and uptake modest, leading to potential inequalities in sexual health.

Paediatrics

Child health surveillance

There have been four editions of the Hall Report, *Health for all Children*.

- The first edition set out a programme of routine reviews for all pre-school children.

- The second edition suggested how this may be delivered.

- The third edition was a response to evolving professional perceptions of preventative healthcare, coupled with rapid changes in the political context in which that care is provided (1996).

- The fourth report adds to the emphasis of health promotion and moves away from a medicalised model of screening.

In September 2003, the Green Paper *Every Child Matters* was published, highlighting the need to maximise opportunity, minimise risk and support children to be healthy, safe, make a positive contribution and achieve economic wellbeing. It sets out the strategy for child health promotion. This report was followed by *Every Child Matters: the next steps* in March 2004, which started to set out the plan for delivery. In September 2004, the National Service Framework for Children, Young People and Maternity Services was launched (www.doh.gov.uk). It comprises 11 standards. The first five apply to all children, Standards 6 to 10 apply to children in special circumstances, and Standard 11 is for maternity services.

- Standard 1: Promoting health and well being, identifying needs and intervening early.
- Standard 2: Supporting parenting.
- Standard 3: Child, young person and family-centred services.
- Standard 4: Growing up into adulthood.
- Standard 5: Safeguarding and promoting the welfare of children and young people.
- Standard 6: Children and young people who are ill.
- Standard 7: Children and young people in hospital.
- Standard 8: Disabled children, young people and those with complex health needs.
- Standard 9: The mental health and psychological wellbeing of children and young people.
- Standard 10: Medicines for children and young people.
- Standard 11: Maternity services.

The Child Health Promotion Programme replaces the current Child Health Surveillance Programme and includes:

- the assessment of the child's and the family's needs
- health promotion
- childhood screening
- immunisations
- early interventions to address identified needs.

The table below sets out an overview of health promotion services that will be offered.

Screening

It is important to make parents aware that screening tests are just that: screening tests. If they have any worries or concerns they need to seek advice from their GP or health visitor.

Age	Intervention
Soon after birth	General physical examination with emphasis on heart, eyes and hips. Administration of vitamin K. BCG and hepatitis B vaccinations in high-risk babies
5–6 days old	Blood spot test for hypothyroidism and phenylketonuria. Sickle cell and cystic fibrosis screening are also being implemented
New birth visit	This is usually around 12 days and done by the health visitor or midwife. As well as assessing the family's needs, they are also given the personal child health record and the 'Birth to Five' guide
6–8 weeks	Physical examination and administration of first set of immunisations: polio, diphtheria, tetanus, whooping cough, Hib and meningitis C
3 months	Second set of immunisations
4 months	Third set of immunisations
By 12 months	Further developmental assessment
Around 13 months	Immunisation against measles, mumps and rubella
2–3 years	Health visitor performs further developmental assessment
3–5 years	Further immunisation against MMR, polio, diphtheria, tetanus and whooping cough
4–5 years	A review at school entry (usually by the school nurse). The foundation stage profile assessment by the child's teacher to look at development of physical, emotional, social and creative development, as well as communication, language and literacy
10–14 years	BCG vaccination given to those who require it. Tetanus, diphtheria and polio boosters (age 13–18 years)

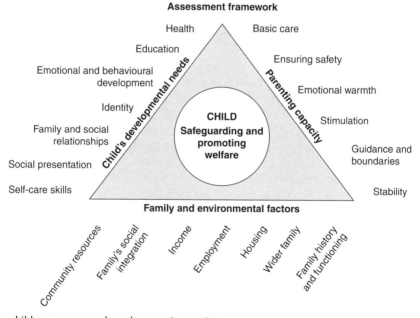

NSF for children, young peole and maternity services.

Developmental dysplasia of the hip

This is a spectrum of conditions where the head of the femur is partly or completely displaced from the acetabulum.

Risk factors include family history, breech presentation, oligohydraminos, postural deformities of the feet, first born, Caesarean delivery and female gender. The incidence is 1.25 in 100 births.

Early detection and conservative treatment are often successful and avoid the need for surgery. Routine screening (Ortalani and Barlow) (valid up to 3 months) misses up to 70% of cases. This is a falsely reassuring 'screening test' for both parents and doctors. Some European countries now have a universal ultrasound screening programme. The UK targets babies with risk factors or with a positive Ortalani or Barlow, aiming for an ultrasound scan by 8 weeks.

Ultrasonography in screening for developmental dysplasia of the hip in newborns: systematic review
BMJ 2005; 330: 1413–15

A total of 188 studies were selected for full assessment, of which 10 met the inclusion criteria for analysis. There were three important findings. First, there is insufficient evidence for the use of ultrasound as a screening tool; second, ultrasound is likely to increase treatment rates, possibly unnecessarily; and finally, the duration of intervention was likely to be lowered by ultrasound screening.

Screening for hearing defects

- Around 840 children each year are born with permanent hearing impairment.

- Around 50% are not diagnosed until they are 18 months old.

- Around 25% are not diagnosed until they are 3 years old (i.e. the distraction test does not pick up some children early enough).

Permanent hearing impairment impacts on communication skills, educational attainment and quality of life. If there is intervention by 6 months, the outcome for all of the above as well as the cost to society, is improved.

Following the Government announcement of the National Newborn Hearing Programme all babies are screened within 48 hours of birth where possible. This is called *otoacoustic emissions testing*. It has been known since the 1970s that for each sound heard by the ear, the ear produces a tiny corresponding sound ('echo') known as otoacoustic emission. This can now be measured by a computer and used clinically. Absence, or a barely audible, echo indicates the child has a hearing problem. Sensitivity is in the range of 80–90%, and costs are less than the distraction tests previously performed at 8 months.

Universal neonatal hearing screening versus screening as part of the management of childhood deafness
Cochrane Database Syst Review 2005; (2): CD003731

Although a number of factors increase the risk of hearing impairment (low birthweight, prematurity, perinatal hypoxia, jaundice, etc.), it can occur without any of these being present. This review of randomised controlled trials looked at the long-term effectiveness of a universal neonatal screening and early treatment programme for hearing impairment with (a) screening and treatment of only high-risk neonates, and (b) opportunistic screening and treatment. It concluded that the evidence for long-term effectiveness of universal screening was not established, and that there need to be ongoing trials to clarify the issue.

Vaccination programme

www.immunisation.nhs.uk

The immunisation schedule has saved more lives than any other public health measure (apart from the provision of clean water). The success of a vaccine is not the number of primary cases of the disease but the number of secondary cases generated from each primary infective source. Please see table on p. 121 for ages recommended for each vaccination.

Measles, mumps and rubella (MMR)

Although the ongoing surveillance has discredited the link with autism and Crohn's disease, this is an emotive topic for all parents. The single vaccines are not licensed for use in the UK (other than rubella). If a single vaccine is requested, it must be done on a named patient basis and be approved by the Medicines Control Agency. The website www.mmrthefacts.nhs.uk is an excellent reference site, and gives direct links to other sites and evidence.

Is the MMR linked to autistic spectrum disorder and Crohn's disease

The first signs of autism generally appear in the second year of life, which co-incides with the MMR vaccination. The incidence is unknown, but is thought to be increasing, as awareness and diagnostic criteria have changed over recent years. Autism has never been linked with the measles vaccine. The questions around the vaccine arose with the introduction of mumps and rubella to produce a triple vaccine. A small number of doctors thought there may be a causative link. A recent Danish trial has upheld the judgement that there is no evidence of a link between MMR and autism.

The MMR scare from 1998 resulted in a 4% drop in uptake, reducing immunisation uptake to 85%. To eliminate measles there needs to be an uptake of 94–96%.

Ileal-lymphoid-nodular hyperplasia, non-specific colitis, and pervasive developmental disorder in children
Lancet 1998; 351:637–41

This paper describes colitis with autism-like behaviour in 12 children. In eight of the children, the parents remembered that symptoms started soon after they received the MMR vaccination. An author went on to recommend that the vaccine should be given as separate antigens at yearly intervals, as the evidence for the MMR was very thin at the time of the issuing of its product licence. This study was published at the start of a very damaging time for the immunisation programme, and a reduction in the uptake of MMR being offered was seen. It is worth noting the study size is 12. There have been 13 million people vaccinated in the UK, and 250 million vaccinations worldwide.

Vaccine for measles, mumps and rubella in children
Cochrane Database Syst Rev 2005; (4): CD004407

Following the search for comparative prospective and retrospective trials, a total of 31 articles were included in the review having satisfied the inclusion criteria. It concluded that exposure to MMR was unlikely to be associated with Crohn's disease, ulcerative colitis or autism. It is likely to be associated with benign thrombocytopenia, parotitis, joint complaints and febrile convulsions within 2 weeks of the vaccination. Although adverse events cannot be separated from its role in the prevention of disease, the authors felt that reporting of safety outcomes had been largely inadequate.

A survey of UK parental attitudes to MMR vaccine and trust in medical authority
Vaccine 2005; Sept 9

This postal survey of 996 parents (both refusing and accepting MMR vaccination for their children) found that parents were supportive of immunisation, but there were high levels of concern about safety in both groups. The findings suggest that a practitioner's advice could be undermined if the Government were to promote the vaccine directly to parents.

MMR vaccine and the incidence of autism recorded by GPs: a time-trend analysis
BMJ 2001; 322: 460–3

This study shows that the increasing incidence of autism has continued over the past decade. If MMR was the cause, a plateau would have been expected, but this has not happened. This paper provides evidence for the view that there is not a causal association between MMR and risk of autism. It concludes that an explanation for the marked increase in the rise of diagnosis of autism in the past decade remains uncertain. A 2005 Japanese study had similar findings.

MMR litigation
The High Court has said that 'no positive link has ever been established' and the Medical Research Council has confirmed this. Judges have gone on to say that 'unsubstantiated health scares endanger children and enrich lawyers'.

The Joint Committee on Vaccination and Immunisation is an independent group that was set up in 1963 to advise Government on matters relating to communicable diseases preventable through immunisation. Its role continues.

Thiomersal in vaccines

Thiomersal is a mercury-based antimicrobial preservative that is found in some DTP preparations (and some Hib vaccines outside the UK). Again this has caught media attention because of suspected links with autism.

It has never been part of live vaccines (MMR and BCG). The theoretical concerns are that in combination, the cumulative mercury dose could exceed recommended safety levels.

The US and Europe regulatory bodies have recommended that it is phased out. This has been endorsed by the World Health Organization, which has also stressed that if thiomersal-free vaccines are not available, vaccination programmes should not be compromised (i.e. children should still be vaccinated).

Three DPT vaccinations with or without Hib would give a maximum cumulative dose of 75 μg ethlymercury – less than half of the 187 μg dose that causes concern. This is cleared quickly and is not cumulative.

A thiomersal and vaccine fact sheet can be found at www.doh.gov.uk.

Autism

Autism is a lifelong developmental disability affecting social and communication skills with varying degrees of severity on a somatic–pragmatic scale. Onset is usually by the age of 3 years, but can go undiagnosed. Early diagnosis enables behavioural therapy, facilitated communication and educational techniques to be introduced, hopefully improving the long-term outcome.

Early identification of autism by the Checklist for Autism in Toddlers (CHAT)
J Roy Soc Med **2000; 93: 521–5**

This is a screening tool that can be used at the 18-month check by GPs or health visitors.

Checklist for Autism in Toddlers

Section A

1	Does your child enjoy being swung, bounced on your knee etc.?	Yes/No
2	Does your child take an interest in other children?	Yes/No
3	Does your child like climbing on things (e.g. stairs)?	Yes/No
4	Does your child enjoy playing peek-a-boo/hide and seek?	Yes/No
5	**Does your child ever pretend, for example, to make a cup of tea using a toy cup and teapot, or pretend other things?**	**Yes/No**
6	Does your child ever use his/her index finger to point to *ask* for something?	Yes/No
7	**Does your child ever use his/her finger to point to indicate interest in something?**	**Yes/No**
8	Can your child play properly with small toys (e.g. bricks, cars) without just mouthing or fiddling with them?	Yes/No
9	Does your child ever bring objects over to show you something?	Yes/No

Section B

1 During the appointment has the child made eye contact with you?   Yes/No
2 **Get child's attention and then point across the room at an**   **Yes/No**
   interesting object and say 'Oh look! There's a [name the toy]'.
   Does the child look across and see what you are pointing at?
3 **Get the child's attention then give him/her a toy cup and teapot**   Yes/No
   and say 'Can you make a cup of tea?' Does the child pretend to
   make or drink the tea?
4 **Say to the child 'Where is the light?'. Does the child point?**   **Yes/No**
5 Can the child build a tower of bricks? (how many?)   Yes/No

If the items in bold print are absent at 18 months, then the child is at high risk for a social communication disorder. If 'No' is the response to all five questions in bold, then the child is at high risk.

A 12-point autism check list is in the process of being validated, it is not dissimilar to the questionnaire above but is based on a scoring system.

Attention deficit hyperactivity disorder (ADHD)

Hyperactivity affects 1–2% of children. There are both ICD-10 and DSM-IV classifications in use. The consequences can be far-reaching, affecting education and causing behavioural problems and social isolation. Benefits can be obtained with medication, behavioural therapy and educational support. Dietary supplements such as flax oil, vitamin C and omega-3 are receiving a lot of attention, and there is anecdotal evidence for excluding some colourings and preservatives.

Access to treatment is influenced by both the parents and the GP. It can lead to conflict, misunderstanding and dissatisfaction if parents' concerns are not taken seriously.

Current research is focusing on cognitive processing, genetic factors, brain function abnormalities and the significance of co-morbidity factors.

Attention-deficit hyperactivity disorder
Lancet 2005; 366(9481): 237–48

This review estimates that this disorder of inattention and impulsivity and hyperactivity can affect up to 12% of children worldwide, and that at least half of the children affected will have impairing symptoms into adulthood. It also considers treatment with methylphenidate and amphetamine to be effective, as well as targeted psychosocial treatments.

NICE Guidelines for methylphenidate for ADHD, October 2000

- Methylphenidate is a sympathomimetic amine that works on dopamine receptors.

- It is used as part of the comprehensive treatment programme (paediatric and psychiatric).

- It is not licensed for children under 6 years, or in cases of thyrotoxicosis or tics.

- Continued prescribing and monitoring may be performed by GPs under a shared-care agreement.

NICE is developing guidance on ADHD: pharmacological and psychological interventions in children.

Sudden infant death syndrome

The confidential enquiry into maternal and child health published its most recent findings for 2000 to 2003 in April 2005 (www.cemach.org.uk/).

Deaths due to sudden infant death syndrome seem to have reduced slightly from 2000 to 2003, but still account for 22% of deaths from birth to 12 months (less in the neonatal period, where up to 50% of deaths are due to immaturity and 22% to congenital malformations).

Risk factors in the infant include the following:

- low birth weight

- prematurity

- gender (60% of cases are boys)

- multiple births

- high birth order (parity).

Risk factors in parents for sudden infant death of their child include the following:

- young maternal age

- unmarried mothers

- maternal smoking in pregnancy

- *smoking after birth* – this increases the risk by fivefold, and is the biggest risk.

Environmental risk factors include:

- low socioeconomic class

- sleeping prone (the Back to Sleep campaign was launched in 1994)

- winter

- overheating

- used cot mattresses (this is being considered in more detail).

Recent data suggest that babies who sleep with a dummy have a reduced risk of cot death.

Babies with parents: case controlled study of factors influencing the risk of SIDs
BMJ 1999; 319: 1457–62

This study looked at 325 deaths (with 1,300 controls). Sharing a bed was not a risk factor but became so when associated with smoking, tiredness, alcohol consumption, overcrowding or thick duvets, especially if the infant was under 14 weeks old.

It is estimated that up to 20% of SIDs involve child abuse. Covert video-recording has increased awareness. However, it raises many medicolegal issues, especially when it is going to be submitted as evidence in court.

CONI (Care of the Next Infant) and the Foundation for the Study of Infant Deaths have been established to support parents. They provide counselling and apnoea alarms, as well as many other resources.

Ophthalmology

Age-related macular degeneration (ARMD)

This is the most common cause of blind registration in industrialised countries. It impairs central vision and progresses slowly over a period of years. There is no cure. There are up to 300,000 cases in the UK (2001 figures) and an increase of 7% is forecast by 2008.

Legal blindness is vision <20/200 (6/60). This means a person can see 20 feet (6 metres) when a normally sighted person could see 200 feet (60 metres).

Dry ARMD is the most common form (85–90% of cases). It is gradual in onset and caused by drusen (thickening of Bruch's membrane between the retina and the choroids) and atrophy of retinal pigment epithelium. Around 15% of cases of dry ARMD will progress to the exudative form.

Wet (or exudative) ARMD accounts for 10% of cases but up to 90% of sight loss in ARMD. It occurs as new blood vessels growing behind the retina leak blood and fluid, causing damage and more rapid loss of vision. This form of ARMD is amenable to treatment with photodynamic therapy or argon laser.

In photodynamic therapy with verteporfin dye, a non-thermal laser activates the dye once it has been injected to close the new choroidal vessels (in exudative/wet ARMD). This treatment looks promising. There is no real evidence for radiotherapy or submacular surgery.

Possible protective factors for the prevention of ARMD

Although you cannot modify age, sex (men are seen to be at greater risk) or genetics (yet), the following factors have been found to be of importance.

- Lifestyle changes
  - wearing sunglasses and brimmed hats in bright light
  - stopping smoking (smoking reduces antioxidant levels) which can more than double the ARMD risk

– nutrition – increase intake of carotenoid-rich vegetables (green leafy vege-tables). Lutein and zeaxanthin are the carotenoids found in the macula, and are thought to be of most importance. A low-fat diet and a healthy approach to food underpin the general principles.

● Statins have now been largely discounted, but it was thought that they may help by reducing cholesterol levels (preventing deposition in Bruch's membrane), through antioxidant properties and by inhibiting endothelial cell apoptosis.

Cholesterol-lowering drugs and risk of age related maculopathy: prospective cohort study with cumulative exposure measurements
BMJ 2003; 324: 255–6

This Dutch study with 26,781 person-years' follow-up found no association between cholesterol-lowering drugs and age-related maculopathy. The authors discussed the fact that previous studies had low statistical powers.

● Regular eye tests would identify eye problems (2-yearly tests are free to people over 60 years of age).

ENT

ENT is one of the largest components of primary care. We manage acute problems, but recurrent and chronic problems are often referred. Although there is now a good evidence base for the more common ailments, it isn't quite as straightforward as it may seem.

Sore throat

This is the most common, overtreated, controversial and mundane (or is it?) symptom in general practice. Symptoms last for up to 10 days and may be associated with systemic features such as fever, malaise and vomiting.

A Cochrane Review looked at antibiotics and complications of sore throats, and concluded that antibiotics offered a small clinical benefit. They were found to reduce the risk of rheumatic fever by up to 30%, but this would be barely significant in the Western world. The incidence of acute otitis media was reduced by 25%.

NICE Referral practice, May 2000 (under pilot)

In recurrent episodes of acute sore throat in children aged up to 15 years, the following should be considered.

● Outcomes are likely to be improved if the parent, child and health professional decide on a treatment in partnership. Communication is key.

● Agree on analgesia that can be used (ibuprofen and/or paracetamol).

- Avoid prescribing antibiotics if acceptable (children issued antibiotics may be at increased risk of further infection and attend more frequently).

- Issue antibiotics if there are:
  - features of systemic upset
  - peritonsillar cellulites
  - a history of rheumatic fever
  - increased risk from infection (e.g. a child with immunodeficiencies or diabetes mellitus).

- A specialist referral should be considered:
  - acutely if there is suspicion of a quinsy, airway obstruction or swelling causing dehydration
  - routinely if there is a history of sleep apnoea, failure to thrive, five or more episodes of infection in the last 12 months (Paradise criteria) or they have guttate psoriasis caused by recurrent tonsillitis.

A quinsy might be more common in unwell patients with three out of four Centor criteria (fever, purulent tonsils, tender cervical nodes and no cough). The incidence has been seen at 1 in 60 if these criteria are met, compared to 1 in 400 when the patient is not systemically unwell. It is worth offering antibiotics to patients who have been unwell for 48 hours and fit the Centor criteria.

Lemierre's syndrome: a forgotten complication of oropharyngeal infection
J Ayub Med Coll Abbottabad 2005; 17(1): 30–3

Apparently *Fusobacterium necrophorum* is the usual aetiological agent which may rarely complicate oropharyngeal infection as septicaemia, septic thrombophlebitis of the internal jugular vein and metastatic lesions (usually in the lungs). In this study of 156 patients admitted with oropharyngeal infection, two (1.28%) patients had features suggestive of Lemierre's syndrome. This will undoubtedly be even more rare in the UK, but the authors conclude that the widespread use of antibiotics significantly reduced incidence of this potentially fatal infection. Recognition, early diagnosis and prolonged treatment with appropriate antibiotics are usually curative.

Acute otitis media

- Around 66% of cases are due to *Haemophilus influenzae* and *Streptococcus pneumoniae*.

- Around 25% of cases are sterile (no organism can be isolated).

- About 10–20% are due to *Mycoplasma* and anaerobes.

- About 4% are viral (although titres are raised in 25%, possibly preceding bacterial infection).

Use of antibiotics for otitis media

Several meta-analyses have shown that the effectiveness of antibiotics is limited in terms of clinical improvement. The advantages of antibiotics include the following:

- there is a bacterial aetiology
- they are cheap and relatively safe
- there is a reduction in complications (e.g. mastoiditis)
- use can reduce symptoms more quickly.

The disadvantages include:

- the cost escalates when you consider prescribing in mass numbers
- they may discourage natural immunity
- they may promote drug resistance
- they may promote dependence on doctors by prescribing.

A randomized, double-blind placebo-controlled non-inferiority trial of amoxicillin for clinically diagnosed otitis media in children 6 months to 5 years of age *CMAJ* 2005; 172(3): 335–41

This study randomly assigned 512 children, aged 6 months to 5 years, with otitis media to receive either amoxicillin (60 mg/kg daily) or placebo for 10 days. Follow-up was on days 1, 2 and 3, and for a final time between days 10 and 14. At 14 days, 84.2% of children receiving placebo and 92.8% of children receiving amoxicillin had clinical resolution of symptoms. More pain and fever were seen in the placebo group in the first two days. There was no difference in recurrence rates by 3 months. The cure rates are not substantially worse in the placebo group than the treatment group.

One of the questions we need to ask is whether we are justified in withholding antibiotics when we know that they improve symptoms in children, especially in those who have systemic symptoms and those who are too young to express their symptoms, especially of pain.

Otitis media with effusion (glue ear)

This is the most common cause of conductive hearing loss in children aged 2–5 years. By the age of 4 years, up to 80% of children will have been affected with it at some time. Hearing loss has knock-on effects to speech development, school performance in writing and spelling, and behaviour (which may be over-boisterous or clingy).
   Around 50% of cases resolve spontaneously within 3 months, and 95% within 12 months.
   Risk factors for developing otitis media with effusion (OME) include:

- passive smoking (environmental tobacco smoke)
- children attending day care (due to transmission rates of infection)
- bottle feeding (breastfeeding may offer some preventative benefits)
- rhinitis, asthma and reflux.

Does passive smoking affect the outcome of grommet insertion in children
J Laryngol Otol 2005; 119(6): 448–54

In this study, 606 children (with 1,174 ears) who underwent grommet insertion were followed up until the grommets were extruded. The median survival rate for grommets was 59 weeks in children who were exposed to passive smoking and 86 weeks for non-exposed children. The extrusion rate was 36% higher at the end of 1 year if both parents smoked compared to the non-smoking group. Postoperative infection rates, attic retraction, post-extrusion myringosclerosis and permanent perforations were more common in children exposed to passive smoking.

Grommets (ventilation tubes) for hearing loss associated with otitis media with effusion in children
Cochrane Database 2005; (1): CD001801

This review was to assess the effectiveness of grommet insertion compared to myringotomy or non-surgical treatment in children with OME. The outcomes studied were hearing level, duration of middle-ear effusion, wellbeing and prevention of sequelae attributable to hearing loss. The authors conclude that an initial period of watchful waiting is appropriate. There is no evidence available for subgroups of children with speech and language delays or learning problems. The dramatic improvements following grommet insertion are usually only seen in the short term.

Gastric reflux in children can mean that gastric juices reflux, via the Eustachian tube, into the middle ear. This can cause inflammation and ideal conditions for secondary infection.

Back pain

- Around 60–80% of the population will have back pain at some point in their life.

- Up to 90% of acute episodes resolve in 6 weeks; if it persists for 12 weeks or more it is a chronic problem.

- Around 7% of people consult their GP each year with back pain.

- A total of 120 million work days/year are lost as a result of back pain.

Diagnosis and management

Red Flags are symptoms and conditions that require urgent imaging, blood tests and referral. They include the following.

- A past medical history of carcinoma, TB, drug abuse or HIV (cause of immunosupression and infection).

- Previous prescription drug use (e.g. steroids).

- Symptoms of night sweats, fever and loss of weight.

- A new structural deformity (e.g. kyphosis) suggestive of fracture.
- Widespread neurology:
  - cauda equina symptoms – these need immediate referral as there is a risk of permanent damage and incontinence. These symptoms include:
    - loss of sphincter control
    - bilateral neurological leg pain
    - saddle loss of sensation.

Patients with simple back pain or isolated nerve root irritation can be managed conservatively. Multilevel or progressive neurological problems require urgent referral.

Clinical Evidence gives a comprehensive outline of current trials for each modality of treatment (www.clinicalevidence.com). Advice includes:

- simple analgesia regularly
- take regular exercise as soon as the pain allows.

Randomized controlled trial of exercise for low back pain: clinical outcomes, costs and preferences
BMJ **1999; 319: 279–83**

This study showed that early access to a doctor (within 3 days) and physiotherapist (within 1 week) for exercise for new-onset back pain was associated with good outcome. Early mobilisation increases the speed of recovery, reduces the length of time off work and reduces the number of recurrences.

- muscle relaxants may help if there is a degree of spasm unresponsive to analgesia
- physiotherapy
- complementary therapy: chiropractic, osteopathy and acupuncture may all be beneficial, although there are no randomised trials confirming this.

Use of complementary and alternative therapies by patients with self-reported chronic back pain: a nationwide survey in Canada
Joint Bone Spine **2005; Sept 7**

Complementary and alternative medicines (CAM) use was associated with younger age, being married, having a higher level of education and earning a higher salary. Overall, CAM users were more active, healthier and had a more involved social life.

Osteoarthritis

Around 20–25% of visits to GPs relate to the musculoskeletal system. Most of these cases are secondary to osteoarthritis. Osteoarthritis, by definition, cannot be cured.

Management

Diet

Other than weight loss, specific diets have no role to play in the management of osteoarthritis and rheumatic conditions. There are reports of vitamin C reducing rates of progression, and improvements with certain seeds and cod liver oil.

Exercise and physiotherapy

Exercise improves muscular tone and joint function, so should not be avoided. Physiotherapy reduces pain and improves joint range and muscle strength, as well as improving mobility and independence.

Home-based exercise programme for knee pain and knee osteoarthritis: randomised controlled trial
BMJ 2002; 325: 752–5

This trial found that simple home exercises can significantly reduce knee pain over a 2-year period.

Glucosamines

These are available as a dietary supplement, which is expensive. There is an option to prescribe on an FP10 (at a dose of 1500 mg/day).

Glucosamine sulphate is a natural substance that forms proteoglycans (part of the articular cartilage). It is thought to be chondro-protective.

Glucosamine long-term treatment and the progression of knee osteoarthritis: systematic review of randomized controlled trials
Ann Pharmacother 2005; 39(6): 1080–7

This study found that there was a large evidence base showing that glucosamine sulphate was more effective than placebo at delaying structural progression in osteoarthritis of the knee. The risk of disease progression was reduced by 54% ($p = 0.0011$) with an NNT = 9. It was also found to improve pain and function, and caused no more adverse effects than placebo.

Local injections

Intra-articular hyaluronic acid gives symptomatic benefit. This has been confirmed in several randomised controlled trials. The lasting effect is uncertain, as is the benefit compared to steroid injection.

Intra-articular hyaluronic acid for treatment of osteoarthritis of the knee: systematic review and meta-analysis
CMAJ 2005; 172(8): 1039–43

This study included 22 trials published up to April 2004. It concluded that intra-articular hyaluronic acid injection has not been proven to be clinically effective and may be associated with greater risk of adverse events.

Rubifacients

Topical creams and gels are often used by patients, especially when they are unable to tolerate systemic treatments. This is often an area targeted in prescribing budgets because of relative lack of evidence and associated costs.

Systematic review of topical rubifacients containing salicylates for the treatment of acute and chronic pain
BMJ 2004; 328: 995–8

This study looked at randomised double-blind trials comparing rubifacients with placebo, all of which were fairly small in number. The conclusion was cautious, but probably indicates that topically applied rubifacients containing salicylates are effective in treating acute pain. At best the NNT is 5.3 (relative benefit 1.5; 95% CI 1.3–1.9).

Complementary therapies

These are all used regularly in subgroups of the population with good effect. Specific randomised trials are lacking.

COX-2 inhibitors

- Around 15% of people on long-term NSAIDs develop ulcers, accounting for 2,000 deaths per year.

- In 1999, more than £170 million was spent on NSAIDs, not including the co-prescribing of gastroprotective agents.

- COX-2 inhibitors are as effective as other NSAIDs in reducing inflammation and pain.

NICE guidelines on cyclo-oxygenase inhibitors, 2001
- These drugs are indicated for pain and stiffness in inflammatory arthritis and short-term pain relief in osteoarthritis.

- They are not recommended for routine use.

- They are recommended for those over 65 year of age who are taking other drugs that could cause gastrointestinal side effects (e.g. steroids and anticoagulants), and those patients that have existing gastrointestinal problems.

A holding statement (February 2005) advised us that NICE will be reviewing its advice.
   Rofecoxib (Vioxx) has recently been withdrawn from the market (September 2004) following an increased incidence of stroke and heart disease in patients using these drugs. Current advice on COX-2 inhibitors from the European Medicines Agency is that:

- they are contra-indicated in patients with established ischaemic heart disease

- caution should be exercised in patients with cardiovascular risk factors

- we should use the lowest dose for the shortest time necessary.

Risk of adverse gastrointestinal outcomes in patients taking cyclo-oxygenase-2 inhibitors or conventional non-steroidal anti-inflammatory drugs: population-based nested case-control analysis
BMJ 2005; 331(7528): 1310–16

Cases were taken from 367 general practices contributing to the UK RESEARCH database. There were 9,407 incident cases identified and 88,867 matched controls. Increased risk of adverse gastrointestinal events was associated with COX-2 inhibitors and NSAIDs. After adjustment for confounders the risk remained significantly higher for naproxen (odds ratio 2.12; 95% CI 1.73–2.58), diclofenac (odds ratio 1.96; 95% CI 1.78–2.15) and rofecoxib (odds ratio 1.56; 95% CI 1.30–1.87) but not for current use of celecoxib (odds ratio 1.11; 95% CI 0.87–1.41). They found that use of ulcer-healing drugs removed the risk for adverse gastric events in all groups of NSAIDs except diclofenac, which still had an increased odds ratio (odds ratio 1.49; 95% CI 1.26–1.76).

Meta-analysis of cyclo-oxygenase-2 inhibitors and their effects on blood pressure
Arch Intern Med 2005; 165(5): 490–6

The review looked at 19 studies (involving a total of 45,457 people). Although COX-2 inhibitors and NSAIDs raised systolic and diastolic blood pressure (by 3.8 mmHg and 2.83 mmHg respectively) this was not significantly more than placebo. A further meta-analysis published showed that there was no significant increase in cardiovascular risk with celecoxib.

Osteoporosis

This is defined by the NHS Consensus Development Conference as a 'progressive skeletal disorder characterised by low bone mass and microarchitectural deterioration of bone tissue with a consequent increase in bone fragility and susceptibility to fracture'.
   The WHO definition is as follows.

- Osteoporosis: bone density >2.5 SD below the mean.

- Osteopenia: >1 SD below the mean.

Note that one definition is a pathological process and the other is an arbitrary point on a scale. The T-score criteria were proposed for epidemiological studies to compare populations and for defining thresholds in clinical trials. Unless stated otherwise, the measurements will be from the femoral neck. They were not intended for diagnosis or management decisions in individual cases.

- It is estimated that up to 3 million women in the UK have osteoporosis.

- The prevalence increases from 2% at 50 years to 25% at 80 years (in women).

- Osteoporosis causes over 180,000 fractures per year (mainly wrist, vertebral and hip fractures) in England and Wales.

- It costs the Government £1.5 billion per year (87% of this is due to hip fractures).

- One in five hip fracture patients die within 1 year, and 50% have severely impaired mobility.

- A third of vertebral fractures cause chronic pain (i.e. there is a huge impact on morbidity and mortality).

Risk factors

These include the following:

- postmenopausal women

- early menopause (before 45 years of age, e.g. following a hysterectomy and oophorectomy)

- immobility

- long-term steroid use (it is suggested that this group receives preventative treatment)

- previous fragility fracture

- high systolic BP (higher rate of bone loss)

- secondary causes:
  - alcoholism
  - thyroid problem (hypothyroidism and hyperthyroidism)
  - liver disease
  - malabsorption
  - hypogonadism in men
  - connective tissue disorders (e.g. rheumatoid and systemic lupus erythematosus).

Around 50% of men and 10% of women will have a secondary cause.

Treatment

Monitoring the effect of treatment has usually been done with repeat DEXA scans, after at least 18 months of treatment. However, bone turnover markers (such as P1NP) may be of more use in the short term and are currently being evaluated.

Prevention/lifestyle changes

- Stop smoking, avoid excess alcohol and take regular weight-bearing exercise.

- Fall prevention – assessment of safety in the home can be provided in primary care.

- Protection of sites of high impact. Hip protectors are of proven benefit with up to 50% reduction in some studies (residential care based).

Calcium supplements

- The recommended daily dose is 1 g for people over 50 years of age.

- There is no evidence that calcium reduces fractures unless it is taken with vitamin D.

Vitamin D

- The recommended daily dose of 400 iU is too low for fracture prevention; 800 iU would usually be used.

- Two trials have shown that vitamin D and calcium reduced risk of fracture by up to 50% over 5 years.

Bisphosphonates

These are now first choice in management of osteoporosis. A once-monthly preparation, ibandronate, has recently been released.

Strontium ranelate

This is a dual agent (like teriparatide) that improves bone mineral density by increasing bone formation and reducing bone resorption.

Hormone replacement therapy

A meta-analysis suggests that this yields a relative risk reduction of 40% (for fractures). However, the benefits are lost within 5 years of stopping HRT. This is a treatment option that is no longer recommended for treatment or prevention because of the risk-factor profile.

Tibolone (bleed-free preparation of HRT)

This has been shown to increase bone mass density in the spine over 2 years.

Selective oestrogen-receptor modulators (e.g. raloxifene)

These decrease the fracture rate by 30% over 3 years at best.

NICE Osteoporosis – secondary prevention, January 2005

Although guidance for primary prevention is still in development the guidance for use of bisphosphonates, raloxifene and teriparatide (a new parathyroid hormone treatment) in secondary prevention is already drawing a degree of criticism because of how restrictive it is.

The standards are as follows.

- All women over 75 years who have sustained a fracture should be treated for presumed osteoporosis without the need for a DEXA scan.

- All women between 65 and 74 years should be treated if osteoporosis is confirmed by DEXA scan.

- Women younger than 65 years should be treated:
  - if they have a bone mineral density less than −3 SD
  - if they have a bone mineral density of −2.5 SD with one or more additional risk factors (BMI <19 kg/m², a family history of maternal hip fracture <75 years, untreated premature menopause, medical disorders associated with bone loss or conditions associated with prolonged immobility).

For treatment, preferences are the bisphosphonates, with raloxifene as an alternative. Teriparatide should be restricted for use in more severe cases.

Several articles have been published which raise concerns about the guidelines. Below are a number of issues that are often discussed.

- The guidelines are too restrictive and will exclude a lot of people who would benefit from treatment.

- The search omitted a number of European articles, casting doubt on the cost-effectiveness calculations.

- The T-score weighting means that, under the guidelines, patients need to be at a higher risk to qualify for treatment.

- It does not take into account the Royal College of Physicians guidance (2002) that patients on long-term corticosteroids should receive treatment at a T-score of −1.5 SD (−2.5 SD in NICE).

- NICE has now agreed that treatment can be given while awaiting a DEXA scan, due to the long delays. How this would then affect their treatment if after scanning they were found to be just outside the treatment criteria is not clear.

Screening

Fractures occur late and there are no symptoms prior to this. All women over 65 years of age in the USA are screened. However, there is currently no universal policy in the UK. When the NICE document *Osteoporosis – primary prevention* is published, it should address this at some level.

Royal College of Physicians guidelines, 1999

These guidelines suggest that DEXA scanning should be offered to individuals with risk factors, as well as those with a low BMI (<19 kg/m²) and those with a strong family history (despite the Finnish study concluding that genetics were not thought to be important).

Useful information can be obtained from the National Osteoporosis Society (www.nos.org.uk).

Alcohol misuse

- Alcohol is responsible for around 22,000 deaths a year in the UK (15,000 due to chronic disease).

- Alcohol misuse accounts for 150,000 hospital admissions a year.

- Around 7% of the UK population have features of mild alcohol dependence.

- Around 21% of 11- to 15-year-olds drink twice a week (an increase of 4% since 1994).

In men, alcohol consumption >300 g/week is associated with increased blood pressure and risk of stroke. Drinking 1–4 units/day in men and 1–2 units/day in women on 5–6 days of the week appears to be protective against CHD and possibly stroke. Tackling those patients who misuse alcohol and getting them to recognise that they are drinking too much is probably where we as GPs could make the biggest impact.

Brief intervention by a GP can be effective, depending on where your patient is in the cycle of change.

In 2004, the first alcohol needs assessment for England was conducted. The key findings were:

- 38% of men and 16% of women (aged 16–64 years) have an alcohol use disorder (equivalent to 8.2 million people)

- over 50% of these are binge drinkers

- 1.1 million people are dependent on alcohol

- the general practice research database study found low levels of formal identification, treatment and referral of patients with alcohol use problems. GPs identify 1 in 67 males and 1 in 82 females who are harmful drinkers

- there is a large gap between the need for alcohol treatment and access to alcohol treatment (only 5.6% of individuals needing help are receiving it).

The Alcohol Harm Reduction Strategy for England
BMJ 2004; 328: 905–6 (Editorial)

This editorial discusses the strategy and the differences between the interim and final reports, and that there is disappointment that a strategy to reduce any increase in alcohol-related harm doesn't adequately focus on reducing alcohol consumption. The author states that 'the complex relation people have with alcohol and how deeply embedded the use of alcohol is in our culture are not sufficiently acknowledged in the report'.

The strategy will tackle the following areas:

- alcohol-related disorder in towns and city centres (crime and disorder)
- improving treatment and support for people with alcohol problems (identification and treatment)
- clamping down on irresponsible promotions by the industry (supply and industrial responsibility)
- providing better information about the dangers of alcohol (education and communication).

Screening tools

CAGE and AUDIT are the most widely validated methods of screening for alcohol use disorders. CAGE seems to be more popular in the UK.

CAGE questionnaire

- Have you ever felt you should **C**ut down?
- Have you ever been **A**nnoyed by someone criticising your drinking?
- Have you ever felt **G**uilty about your drinking?
- Have you ever had an **E**ye opener (early morning drink) to steady your nerves/get rid of your hangover?

A score of 2 or more has a high correlation with alcoholism, but this screening tool has a low sensitivity and specificity.

AUDIT (Alcohol Use Disorder Identification Test)

This WHO screening tool is thought to be a more suitable screening test for excessive drinking at the less severe end of the spectrum. It has been found to have a higher sensitivity and specificity than the CAGE questionnaire.

FAST

This is another quick screening test. Here, the focus is on the frequency of risky levels of consumption of alcohol, and asking the patient to rate the following:

- how often they drink
- to what extent they drink
- whether a friend or health professional has ever been concerned about the amount they drink.

Effectiveness of treatment for alcohol problems: findings of the randomised UK alcohol treatment trial (UKATT)
BMJ 2005; 331: 541–4

The objective of this trial was to compare social behaviour and network therapy with that of the proven motivational enhancement therapy. Both groups (689 people at 3 months and 617 at 12 months) had reduced alcohol consumption and dependence. The study concluded that the two methods did not differ significantly.

Drug misuse

- It is estimated that 250,000 people in the UK suffer from problems related to drug misuse.

- It is estimated that 20,000 young people become adult problem drug users every year.

- One in 65 intravenous drug users has HIV (1 in 25 in London).

- More than two in five intravenous drug users have been infected with hepatitis C.

Modernising the Health Service looks at drug issues in part, and aims to provide targeted prevention activity for at least 30% of young people most vulnerable to drug misuse.

Guidelines on Clinical Management is a booklet for guidance on drug use and treatment first published in 1984 and is regularly updated (most recently in 1999).

The Home Office recognises the problems caused by drug use, from the health implications through to crime and underachievement in education by young people, and has many initiatives under way.

- Blueprint – this is a 5-year research programme looking at the effectiveness of drug prevention initiatives in school and community settings.

- The Drug Intervention Programme has screened 15,860 young offenders.

- Talk to Frank is a website and helpline for young people (www.talktofrank.com) to find out more information.

- Positive Futures aims to divert young people from drug misuse through sports and art.

There are many other plans through, for example, the National Service Framework for Young People.

The GP's role is primarily identification of patients who have problems and need specialist help. Although there has been an increase in the number of GPs providing specialist care as part of enhanced services and as GPs with special interests, most would still refer patients on. Of equal importance is the recognition of problems such as mental health complications, infections (e.g. HIV and hepatitis) and thrombosis.

Although addicts want GPs to be involved in their treatment, doctors should not be pressurised into accepting responsibilities beyond their level of expertise. This has been brought to our attention most recently by a case in which a GP was charged with manslaughter when one of his teenage patients died of a methadone overdose. An initial thorough assessment is mandatory.

In March 2001, the Department of Health issued a statement on the use of buprenorphine in the treatment of drug addiction. It has been recognised for use in opiate withdrawal, detoxification and maintenance. In randomised trials it has had comparable success to methadone.

Comparison of pharmacological treatments for opioid-dependent adolescents: a randomised controlled trial
Arch Gen Psychiatry **2005; 62(10): 1157–64**

This study looked at treatment with either buprenorphine or clonidine for opioid dependence. A total of 72% of adolescents receiving buprenorphine compared with 39% on clonidine were retained in treatment after 28 days ($p < 0.05$). It concluded that buprenorphine with behavioural intervention was significantly more efficacious.

Obesity

Obesity is defined as a BMI $>30 \, \text{kg/m}^2$.

- Over 20% of men and women in the UK are obese. It is a huge medical, public health and economic problem, with genetic and environmental determinants.
- Around 6% of all deaths can be attributed to obesity (National Audit Office, 2001).

Reducing obesity is one of the six priorities of the *Choosing Health* White Paper. The strategies go beyond the recommendations of the House of Commons Select Committee's Report of May 2005. The Government's response to the report lays out 52 recommendations. It includes the recognition that further data collection is needed, the approach schools should take, the role of OFSTED in assessing these directives, a national walking strategy, the roles of healthcare professionals (pharmacological, surgical, psychological and behavioural aspects), as well as the need for a dedicated framework for obesity building on the current National Service Frameworks. One specific recommendation is that there should be a wide-ranging programme of solutions:

- health promotion
- education about food
- restriction of promotion of unhealthy foods for children
- a comprehensive care pathway on obesity.

Obesity Care Pathway 2005

www.nationalobesityforum.org.uk

This publication offers a toolkit for healthcare professionals and considers the following:

- the need for baseline patient data and investigations

- patient motivation

- healthy eating

- physical activity

- integrated weight-management programmes

- the role of pharmaceuticals.

It highlights the use of waist circumference alongside BMI as an aid to stratifying risk and monitoring success.

Orlistat (Xenical) and sibutramine (Reductil)

NICE has published similar guidelines for the use of both of these drugs. Criteria include a BMI >30 kg/m^2 (>28 kg/m^2 if associated with risk factors). Prior to starting treatment patients need to have lost 2.5 kg over 4 weeks, and once started they need to lose 5% of their body weight over 12 weeks. If this is not achieved treatment should be discontinued.

Treating obesity in individuals and populations
BMJ 2005; 331: 1387–90 (Clinical Review)

This article discusses the fact that most research has given us information on what doesn't work in treating obesity, but very little has given us specific answers on what does work. It acknowledges that the effectiveness of lifestyle interventions is limited, and that the emphasis should now be on public health measures and pharmacological approaches.

Comparison of the Atkins, Ornish, Weight Watchers and Zone diets for weight loss and heart disease risk reduction. A randomised controlled trial
JAMA 2005; 293: 43–53

The investigators enrolled and randomised 160 adults (mean BMI 35) with known dyslipidaemia, hypertension or fasting hyperglycaemia. The drop-out rate was 42% by 12 months, the most common reason being that the diet was too hard to follow. In each group, 25% sustained a 5% weight loss and 10% a loss of 10% of initial body weight at 1 year. Improvement in cardiac risk factors was directly proportional to the amount of weight lost, and was similar among the diet groups. The study concluded that all diets were successful – the key is patient motivation and self-selection of the diet that suits them best.

Prognosis in obesity (we all need to move a little more and eat a little less)
BMJ 2005; 330: 1339–40 (Editorial)

A fantastic title that really says it all. This discussion touches on lots of points, most topically the 2004 White Paper *Choosing Health* and the subsequent action plan

Choosing a Better Diet, which have both set tough targets to reduce childhood obesity. Both sides of the energy-balance equation must be tackled and are well within the range of day-to-day variability in activity and diet.

Exercise

Active adults live longer!

Obesity in the UK, both in children and adults, is increasing. This has numerous implications for health (non-insulin dependent diabetes mellitus, coronary heart disease, osteoarthritis, etc.). Exercise is effective for long-term weight reduction/ regulation. The gold standard randomised controlled trials are difficult to perform in terms of blinding.

The White Paper *Choosing Health*, National Service Frameworks and care pathways are some of the documents that touch on the importance of exercise.

Effects on cardiovascular disease

- Exercise reduces primary and secondary cardiovascular disease.
- Coronary heart disease can be reduced by 20–30% in men.
- Stroke could be reduced by 30–40%.
- Blood pressure can be reduced by up to 10 mmHg systolic and 8 mmHg diastolic.
- Exercise increases HDL-cholesterol levels.

Musculoskeletal effects

- Exercise has been shown to increase mobility and reduce falls in the elderly.
- It can reduce the rate of hip fracture by up to 50%.
- If weight-bearing, it can increase bone density.

Psychiatric effects

- Exercise reduces and relieves anxiety.
- It appears to have an antidepressant effect.

Other effects

- Exercise can prevent non-insulin dependent diabetes mellitus (NIDDM) in 25% of cases.
- It improves glucose tolerance in NIDDM.
- People who exercise live longer.
- Graded aerobic exercise improves fatigue, functional capacity and fitness in patients with chronic fatigue syndrome.

The role of the GP and primary care is not clear, in that although we are ideally placed, we lack a strong consensus on how to approach this, which exercise programme would benefit which patient and whether we should be 'prescribing' exercise.

The current advice (from the British Heart Foundation) is 30 minutes of moderate exercise every day (in a healthy adult), although shorter bouts of more physical exercise can give similar benefits.

Exercise on prescription is something to be wary of, as 'prescription' implies a full understanding of the possible side effects and complications. The defence unions have advised against prescribing exercise if you do not have the skill to evaluate the patient. However, you could recommend it.

Part 2

Introduction

General practice has never been more focused on the primary healthcare team and the necessity for teamwork than it is at the moment. Part 2 is dedicated to non-clinical issues, the latest policies, and the more ambiguous topics that may be examined and are worth considering. These topics will become part of your everyday working knowledge. In exam terms, although you need to have an understanding of such issues for the written papers (application of your understanding in formulating your answers shows a difference in the level of candidate being examined), you will be most likely to come across specific questions related to these topics in the oral examination.

A brief history of general practice

The first reference to general practice was around 200 years ago, and since then development has been slow but has created an essentially stable primary healthcare system.

1815	General practice became a recognised profession
1841	Royal Pharmaceutical Society of Great Britain was established
1858	General Medical Council established to control standards and conduct, educate doctors, and protect public and profession from quacks
1911	David Lloyd George set up medical insurance
1920	Dawson Report on the future of primary and secondary care
1942	Beveridge Report on the setting up of a Welfare State
1946	NHS established under Labour Government
1952	College of General Practitioners founded (Royal status granted in 1967)
1966	General Practice Charter – the main principles were better pay, seniority, group practices, designated area allowances, financial recognition of out-of-hours and reimbursement schemes for staff salaries
1968	Recommendation of a three-year vocational training scheme (VTS) by Royal College of General Practitioners; compulsory from 1982
1971	Direct access to laboratory facilities
1990	Government paper *Working for Patients*

- Set performance targets
- Increased percentage income from patient numbers
- New items-of-service payments to encourage minor surgery, child health surveillance, health promotion and deprived-area incentives

The new contract was introduced

1991	Fundholding commenced
1995	General Medical Council's *Good Medical Practice*
1996	White Paper on *Primary Care: delivering the future*
1997	Summative assessment at completion of VTS became mandatory
1998	Primary care groups developed to replace fundholding
2000	NHS Plan
2002	New World Organization of Family Doctors (WONCA) definition of general practice
2004	New general medical services (nGMS) contract
2005	Practice-based commissioning

GMC's *Duties of a Doctor*

- Make the care of your patients your first concern.
- Treat every patient politely and considerately.
- Respect patient dignity and privacy.
- Listen to patients and respect their views.
- Give patients information in a way they can understand.
- Respect patients' rights to be fully involved in decisions about their care.
- Keep professional skills and knowledge up to date.
- Recognise the limits of your professional competence.
- Be honest and trustworthy.
- Respect and protect confidential information.
- Make sure your personal beliefs do not prejudice your patient's care.
- Act quickly to protect patients from risk if you have a good reason to believe you or a colleague may not be fit to practise.
- Avoid abusing your position as a doctor.
- Work with colleagues in the ways that best serve your patients' interests.

In all of the above matters you must never discriminate unfairly against your patients or colleagues. You must always be prepared to justify your actions.

What is a good doctor and how do you make one?
BMJ 2002; 324: 556–710

This is an edition dedicated to good performance and the qualities that contribute to being a good doctor, e.g. contentment. The GMC is in consultation in regard to updating its guidance *Good Medical Practice* (1999). Given the numerous legal cases that have been brought over the past five years it will be interesting to see what changes are felt appropriate.

WONCA European definition of general practice

WONCA is the World Organization of Family Doctors, which published a new definition of family practice in 2002. An overview of this was published in *The New Generalist* in spring 2003.
   The discipline of general practice:

- is normally the first point of medical contact in the healthcare system
- makes efficient use of resources through co-ordination
- develops a person-centred approach

- has a unique consultation process that establishes a relationship over time
- has a decision-making process based on prevalence and incidence of illness
- manages acute and chronic problems
- promotes health and wellbeing
- deals with health problems in their physical, psychological, social, cultural and existential dimensions.

The speciality of general practice was summarised as follows.

- GPs are specialist physicians trained in the principles of discipline. They are primarily responsible for provision of comprehensive and continuing care.
- They care for individuals in the context of their family, community and culture. They recognise that they have a professional responsibility to their community.
- They exercise their professional role by promoting health, preventing disease and providing cure or palliation.
- They must take responsibility for maintaining their skills, personal balance and values.

The future of general practice

Shaping Tomorrow: issues facing general practice in the new millennium

Parliament is responsible for the entire NHS. General practice is here to provide a primary care service to the whole population (i.e. it is the first point of contact with the NHS, together with Accident and Emergency, Family Planning, NHS Direct, genito-urinary clinics, etc.). Everyone in the UK has the right of access to a GP.

Our role is demand led and covers preventative healthcare, acute and chronic diseases, business management, research, audit, training and teaching, as well as co-ordination between services for patients and their families.

Over the past 50 years there have been six major changes:

- in 1948, the NHS was established
- in 1966, the GP Charter was introduced
- in 1990, the new contract was introduced
- in 2000, the NHS Plan was published
- in 2004, the new GMS contract was introduced
- in 2005, practice-based commissioning was introduced.

As part of the ongoing development, a discussion document, *Shaping Tomorrow: issues facing general practice in the new millennium*, was issued by Chris Mihill of the

General Practitioners Committee (GPC) of the BMA. It has collected views from the profession, politicians and patients, addressing topics such as what patients want and what model should replace the 'Dr Finlay icon of the all-purpose, 24-hour, home-visiting family doctor'. There are 12 chapters in the document, from which I have selected and summarised what I consider to be the most important issues.

My doctor or any doctor?

The drive to make speedy access a primary care priority is not necessarily the main concern of patients. Two main patient groups have emerged, namely the essentially well who value easy access to healthcare with staff able to deal with their problems, and those with chronic diseases who prefer to see their own doctor.

Many GPs see the personal relationship with patients as central to what they do, while others view it as a fading asset due to modern-day careers. In many busy urban practices the concept of 'my doctor' is already meaningless, and some feel that the future will be about 'one-hit' consultations.

Interestingly, in countries where there is little continuity of care (or records) there are higher rates of investigation. Here lies an obvious argument for continuity of both care and records.

Should GPs let go and use the primary healthcare team?

This question really focuses on the purpose of the consultation, and although most patients are happy to see a nurse for triage or treatment of a minor illness, there is the flip side of the coin that no consultation is trivial, but rather it is an opportunity for discovering hidden agendas and health promotion. If such points of contact were lost, would the 'holistic care' approach be jeopardised? Would patients view nurse appointments as second class?

Interestingly, although over the past 10 years in the USA nurse care has been dramatically increased, there has not been a reduced demand on doctors. Is this because patient demand is being fuelled? Or is it because doctors are good at dealing opportunistically with problems when the reason for attendance is otherwise trivial? Either way, further cost analyses are needed to determine the overall economic implications of nurse practitioners and whether they really do reduce doctors' workload.

Independent contractor status vs. salaried service

Independent contractor status is deemed to allow GPs greater control over their working practice, hours and staff, and to enable them to act as advocates on behalf of their patients. This is thought to encourage innovation, change and efficiency. This style of contract means that the Government gets more for its money. If GPs were all salaried for certain hours (i.e. 40 hours per week), there would be more doctors needed and consequently more would be spent on wages.

However, there is a widely held belief that independence is an illusion and will become increasingly so in the world of primary care trusts, clinical governance,

National Service Frameworks and the Healthcare Commission. Taking a salaried stance does not mean that you lose your autonomy, or that you can no longer be an advocate for your patient.

The question arises as to whether it is possible to be an independent practitioner without being an independent contractor.

A job for life or a portfolio career?

Women, ethnic doctors and non-principals are underused resources. Young doctors are wanting flexible careers, to work part time, the chance to move between practices or even to mix general practice with other careers. This situation needs to be recognised and addressed to help keep morale high within the profession and stop doctors leaving. Personal medical services (PMS) pilots are exploring these options and are supported nationally (stating the obvious, as this is where the funding is coming from).

Gatekeeper: is there still a role? Will walk-in centres and NHS Direct change the game?

Walk-in centres and NHS Direct have increased the number of access points to primary care. It is anticipated that in the future this, or another form of triage, will be used in the first instance, with GPs further down the line.

Is this a way of tackling the social aspect of modern-day medicine for disbanded families (the grandmother role)? Will GPs be expected to take on specialist roles because they are a cheaper option than secondary care?

GP supporters recognise that we protect patients from unnecessary over-investigation, so by definition are cost saving.

Clinical autonomy: does it have a place any more?

This in a way goes back to the independent contractor status issue in that, whatever your opinion, we live in the world of NICE, National Service Frameworks, guidelines, protocols, evidence-based medicine, the Health Commission and clinical governance.

Does autonomy mean anything any more? The answer is yes, it does. There has to be autonomy. Although there are guidelines, you do not have to follow them if your patient dictates otherwise. The time this will become problematic is when pay or contracts are performance related (audit, etc.). It would have to include these scenarios to account for shortfalls in achievement if this was an issue.

Primary care groups: working together or professional straitjacket?

Primary care groups/trusts mean increasing accountability and increasing pressure to deliver consistent care in an evidence-based way. This is not an easy task – are we compromising our patients by becoming the body for distributing services with an 'essentially inadequate budget'?

Promoting quality: what makes a good GP? Will revalidation stop bad doctors?

This chapter looks at issues such as quality (which in itself will not mean the same to all of us), consistency and increasing the number of GP specialists (i.e. additional GP roles contracted by the primary care trust – patients would then be referred to secondary care from that point).

Future pressures

This looks at what patients want (not necessarily need), funding and rationing. Pressure will come from all areas – the elderly, genetics, the Internet, consumerism and patient expectations – all of which will drive standards.

Clare Raynor of the Patients' Association believes that the way forward is seeing that patients are as much part of the healthcare team as the professionals.

Internationally, general practice in the UK is often regarded as a model of primary care. It is important that it remains so.

Shaping Tomorrow concludes that change is being imposed by the Government (like it or not!) and the challenge is to retain those parts of general practice that hold value and satisfaction for patients and doctors. To do this, we need to define what is special and central to what we do, and then fight to keep it. It is better to try and shape tomorrow rather than have it imposed on us.

As yet it is not clear what the 'Millennium GP' should look like! (Yes, it actually says that!)

NHS Plan

This is a 10-year reform plan/vision for the NHS that was published in July 2000. It outlines a new delivery system for the NHS, with changes for social services and NHS staff groups. While it continues to underpin the founding principles of the NHS (access to care for all on the basis of need, not ability to pay) it will bring about far-reaching changes across the NHS.

There are five main challenges that need to be addressed.

1 *Partnership* – across the NHS to ensure the best possible care.

2 *Performance* – setting and delivering high standards within the NHS.

3 *Professions* – the wider NHS workforce must work together to deliver services for patients, breaking down the traditional barriers.

4 *Patient care* – delivery should be fast and convenient, listening to need and letting patients know their rights.

5 *Prevention* – promoting healthy living across all societies, and tackling variations in care.

In January 2001, the Department of Health published *Primary Care, General Practice and the NHS Plan*, which covered much the same ground, but was aimed more specifically at primary care professionals. I have broken these down into digestible chunks with the initial timescale plans.

Planned investment

Chronic underfunding has been acknowledged, and there is now a plan for sustained increases in funding.
By 2004:

- 6,500 more therapists
- 2,000 more GPs
- 7,500 more consultants
- 20,000 more nurses
- 1,000 more medical student places
- 7,000 extra beds in hospital/intermediate care.

By 2010:

- 100+ new hospitals
- 500 one-stop primary care centres
- 3,000+ GP premises will be modernised.

In addition, childcare support will be available for NHS staff, with 100 on-site nurseries.

Information technology/accessibility

By 2002:

- all GPs will have access to the NHS net.

By 2004:

- access to electronic personal medical patient records (EPR); 75% of hospitals and 50% of primary care trusts and primary healthcare teams will have implemented EPRs
- electronic prescribing of medication
- a single call to NHS Direct will be a one-stop gateway to out-of-hours care.

By 2005:

- electronic booking of appointments (Choose and Book)
- local health services to have provision for telemedicine

- maximum wait no longer than 48 hours for a routine GP appointment or 24 hours to see a practice nurse
- maximum wait for any stage of treatment no longer than 6 months (3 months by 2008).

General practice

By 2001:

- every primary care group must have in place a system to monitor practice referral rates.

By 2002:

- a third of all GPs will be expected to be working to PMS contracts.

By 2003:

- primary care groups will have become primary care trusts
- occupational health services to be extended to GPs and their staff.

By 2004:

- there will be extended nurse prescribing (over 50% will be able to prescribe).

There will be deeper partnerships with the pharmaceutical industry.

Patient involvement

By 2002:

- patient advocates in every trust
- PALS (Patient Advocacy and Liaison Service).

There will also be:

- further overhaul of the complaints system; the NHS will act on concerns before they become complaints
- increased lay input at every level, including advising NICE
- patient views on local health services will help decide how much cash they receive
- letters about patient care will be copied to the patient
- if an operation is cancelled, the patient can choose the date within 28 days or the hospital will pay for it to be done at another hospital of the patient's choosing.

Other points raised

These include the following:

- anti-ageism policy

- nursing care in nursing homes to be free

- better access to dental care

- better diet, with fruit available in schools for 4- to 6-year-olds

- retirement health checks

- modern contracts for doctors

- new care trusts to commission health and social care in a single organisation.

Out-of-hours care/24-hour responsibility

Patient demand for out-of-hours care has been steadily increasing over the past 40 years. This is reflected by the increase in night visits claimed and the attendance in casualty departments. Deputising services and out-of-hours co-operatives have changed the way in which GPs fulfil their 24-hour responsibility to their patients.

Raising Standards for Patients: new partnerships in out-of-hours care was published in October 2000, followed by the 3-year guidance plan. It made various recommendations, including:

- triage through a single call to NHS Direct by 2004 (for all out-of-hours care)

- electronic records which out-of-hours staff can access

- quality assessments of medical staff, organisations and access through clinical governance.

NHS Direct

NHS Direct is a 24-hour telephone advice line staffed by 'specially trained' nurses that aims to empower patients by giving them 'easier and faster information about health, illness and the NHS' (i.e. by going some way towards the Government's vision of a modernised healthcare system). It now allows single-call access to out-of-hours care (the Exemplar programme), offering a triage service, and has been gradually increasing in capacity since 1998.

At present it is mainly being used by patients for reassurance and as an out-of-hours service (72% of calls were made after GP surgeries were closed), and caller satisfaction rates are reported to be high (*Evaluation of NHS Direct First-Wave Sites: first interim report to the DoH*). This report also highlighted that different advice was being offered by different centres for identical 'dummy cases' in the pilot stages of NHS Direct.

Positive points included the following:

- aimed at reducing NHS workload
- easy access for patients
- empowers patients
- encourages self-care
- accompanying NHS Direct healthcare guide.

Concerns include the following:

- may fuel workload/demand
- issues surrounding continuity of care
- missed diagnosis with telephone consultations
- will there be adequate integration with out-of-hours cover? If not this may cause confusion
- not equally accessible to all (e.g. deaf, elderly, mentally ill, non-English speaking).

The NHS Direct healthcare guide has been written by Dr Ian Banks (a GP in Northern Ireland) with the help of an editorial board. The literature is designed to be used in conjunction with NHS Direct. It gives basic information using narratives and flow charts on health and illness, as well as giving a guide as to when patients should contact NHS Direct for further advice. It is available both as a printed booklet and on the Internet (www.nhsdirect.nhs.uk). Again a large problem is promotion and accessibility to those most in need (e.g. socially deprived or illiterate).

To date, NHS Direct has not reduced pressure on the NHS, nor has it appeared to uncover extra demand previously unrecognised. However an analysis in Derbyshire in August 2001 showed that GP workload was eased by 34%.

The National Audit Office's report *NHS Direct in England* found:

- some co-operatives (in the North East) had an 18% drop in calls when callers were transferred to NHS Direct first
- high levels of customer satisfaction.

Impact of NHS Direct on general practice consultations during the winter 1999–2000: analysis of routinely collected data
BMJ 2002; 325: 1397–8

The introduction of NHS Direct had no impact on the number of consultations for influenza-like illness and other respiratory infections. NHS Direct was not introduced to increase or decrease the number of consultations but to make them more appropriate. This was not looked at in the study.

Effect of introduction of integrated out-of-hours care in England: observational study
BMJ 2005; 331: 81–4

This study aimed to quantify service integration achieved in the national Exemplar programme for single-call access to out-of-hours care through NHS Direct and its effect on the wider healthcare system. Outcomes measured were extent of integration, impact on ambulance transport, attendance at Accident and Emergency, minor injury units, walk-in centres and emergency admissions to hospitals. It concluded that most patients made two calls to contact NHS Direct and then had to wait for nurse feedback (29% achieved single-call access). Emergency ambulance transports increased in three of the four exemplars. The overall concern was the lack of capacity within NHS Direct to support the National Implementation Strategy.

Walk-in centres

These have been developed to cover part of the demand for out-of-hours care, to offload some of the burden on Accident and Emergency departments, to improve access to healthcare professionals and to help reduce GP workload by providing treatment for and information about minor conditions.

As with NHS Direct, walk-in centres have been subject to the criticism that they have not undergone formal assessment. In the initial period, 40 centres were opened in England. The *King's Fund Report* released at the end of 2001 called for a halt in the expansion of the pilot programme and highlighted the need for more skills training for nurses and for improved links with GPs and other healthcare providers.

When trying to determine the efficacy of walk-in centres it is worth bearing in mind that:

- they direct funds from other areas of primary care

- there can be a lack of continuity of care

- the service may generate a new demand.

An observational study comparing quality of care in walk-in centres with GPs and NHS Direct using standardised patients
BMJ 2002; 324: 1556–9

This looked at five clinical scenarios: postcoital contraception, chest pain, sinusitis, headache and asthma. Walk-in centres performed adequately and safely compared to GPs and NHS Direct for the above conditions. Impact of referrals on the workload of other healthcare providers was deemed to need further research.

Effect of NHS walk-in centre on local primary healthcare services: before and after observational study
BMJ 2003; 326: 530–2

This study looked at the effect of a walk-in centre in Loughborough on local primary and emergency services. Market Harborough was used as the control town. It found that the workload of GPs was not greatly affected. However, the minor injuries unit (attached to the walk-in centre) had a significant increase in workload.

Intermediate care

'Intermediate care' is a new phrase for the old concept of bridging the gap between primary and secondary care. This is not just about providing social care for elderly patients in the effort to free hospital beds, but can also encompass various schemes, such as mental health, the young chronically ill, etc. It should not be regarded as a cheap alternative to acute hospital and specialist care.

Intermediate care, by definition, is not part of the current GP contract/GMS services. Although much of the medical input is provided by GPs, it does not follow that if no GP cover is available these patients should be allocated to a GP until they are discharged from their intermediate care bed. It is envisaged that intermediate care beds will primarily be nurse managed on a day-to-day basis, and GPs would be involved from the diagnostic, management and review aspect. The role of community matrons as part of the intermediate care team is starting to be explored.

Hospital at home vs. hospital care in patients with exacerbations of COPD: prospective randomised controlled trial
BMJ 2000; 321: 1245–8

There was no difference in readmission rates, lung function or mortality at 3 months when comparing hospital at home to hospitalisation.

Stroke rehabilitation at home
Age and Ageing 2001; 30: 303–10

This study looked at effectiveness and cost of rehabilitation compared to follow-up in a day hospital. In this randomised controlled trial of 480 patients there was no difference in outcome or cost.

For intermediate care/hospital at home to be successful, it is important to set up measurements of success, and to determine the types of patient who are to be cared for and the level of care to be input, as well as determining resource allocation. A new paper, *Intermediate Care and Specialist GPs*, calls for the expansion of the numbers of GPs and nurses with the necessary educational support to cope with what will become an increased demand.

Nurse practitioners

Nurse practitioners are playing an increasingly large part in the service provision of primary care. With the ongoing struggle to fill GP posts in some areas, nurse practitioners will continue to expand their role. Their roles are varied, depending on the skills and experience of the nurse, but the main areas of input are disease prevention, health promotion, chronic disease management, immunisation (child and travel), smears and family planning. Management of minor illnesses, triage and prescribing are areas of ongoing development, but require specific diagnostic skills training to reduce errors in treatment and advice.

From the GP's perspective, this addition to the team will hopefully reduce workload and improve access and satisfaction, as well as standards of care. GPs may have more time for more challenging problems and may be able to operate bigger lists.

Possible problems include the following.

- Nurses are not regulated, so who will be accountable? Will it be us as GPs?

- Is a two-tier system being introduced? Will GP recruitment suffer further because of this, particularly in inner cities?

- We may lose continuity of care as the GP.

- Nurses may misdiagnose rarer but serious conditions if there is no diagnostic index of suspicion.

- GPs may start to lose their generalist role.

- Protocols and guidelines need to be developed. Who will write these? Will it be the GP? Would they then be accountable when the patient dictates a variation from the directive?

- Nurses as a body are already overloaded trying to reach National Service Framework targets, etc. Can we really expand their role further given the current shortfall in number?

- Funding and training as well as interest/staffing are areas where needs have to be met.

Systematic review of whether nurse practitioners working in primary care can provide equivalent care to doctors
BMJ 2002; 324: 819–23

This review concluded that there would be higher levels of patient satisfaction and a high quality of care. It acknowledged the different pressures on nurses and doctors. It pointed out that the trials did not look at missed diagnoses (i.e. long-term follow-up, etc.).

Impact of practice nurses on workload of GPs: randomised controlled trial
BMJ 2004; 328: 927–30

This was a randomised controlled before-and-after trial of 34 general practices in the Netherlands. Five nurses were randomly allocated to practices to undertake specific duties. Workload was derived from 28-day work diaries and measured for 6 months before and 18 months after the introduction of a nurse practitioner. They found that there was no significant difference in workload for GPs in this short term.

Community matrons

These posts are only just being developed and are a logical extension into the community of nurse practitioners. As yet there are no data or trials looking at the effectiveness in terms of their brief.

Their role includes the following.

- To avoid inappropriate hospital admissions.

- To optimise the health and wellbeing of adults who meet set criteria for being managed within their own home, e.g. falls, non-specific illness, long-term conditions, revolving-door patients.

- They will define the category of patient, develop care plans and evaluate progress.

Nurse prescribing

www.doh.gov.uk/nurseprescribing

By 2004, the Government had wanted 10,000 nurse prescribers. The current total is 6,000. This underlines the length of practical and clinical training needed. Once trained, the prescriber has to have signed up, otherwise they would be prescribing illegally.

Prescribing by nurses falls into five categories.

1 *Specific exemptions* (e.g. midwives, health visitors and district nurses).

2 *Patient-specific directives* – a written instruction from a recognised prescriber, which is patient-specific.

3 *Patient group directives* – a named drug can be issued for a specific clinical situation (all must conform with HSC 2000/026). This is as opposed to a clinical management plan, which is patient-specific not drug-specific.

4 *Independent nurse prescribers* – who are deemed competent to assess, diagnose and make treatment decisions, and who may prescribe from the nurse formulary from the *British National Formulary* (for certain conditions).

5 *Supplementary prescribers* – an independent nurse prescriber who has a voluntary prescribing contract working to clinical management plans (patient-specific, with no restriction on the condition). Some pharmacists have undertaken this role.

The benefits of nurse prescribing include:

- it can free up medical time

- the prescription can be written by the clinician who sees the patient

- nurses can work independently

- it improves patient safety. The professional seeing the patient is trained to make the decision and as a doctor signing a script you are reliant on often-inadequate information

- safety is helped by the use of electronic systems that highlight interactions.

The drawbacks include:

- the current nurse prescribing formulary is limited

- it raises issues such as being able to use doxycycline for acne but not for chlamydia

- a number of GP systems will not accept nurse prescribers and scripts must be a hand-written duplicate

- there is concern about the safety fears of many prescribers, drug safety and the necessary continuity of patient care.

Extended prescribing by UK nurses and pharmacists
BMJ 2005; 331: 1154–5 (Editorial)

This was written following the announcement that nurse and pharmacist independent prescribers are now able to prescribe any licensed drug, except controlled drugs. The editorial discusses the safety issues around prescribing, and the fact that although it is an incredibly powerful tool in tackling disease, it is a significant cause of patient harm.

Pharmacists

The role of the pharmacist in primary care is also increasing. Community pharmacists are an underused resource in the NHS, despite their level of training. The Government launched the first wave of its National Medicines Management Programme in October 2001, and this project may help it go some way towards reaching its National Service Framework targets and meeting patient demand.

Following successful pilot studies and with the new pharmacy contract, repeat prescribing (along with other enhanced services such as warfarin monitoring and services for drug misusers) for patients is to be undertaken by pharmacists and commissioned by primary care. Other areas of pharmacist management that will be considered in the future include lipid management, immunisation, diabetes and weight management.

Repeat prescribing: a role for the community pharmacists in controlling and monitoring repeat prescriptions
Br J Gen Pract 2000; 50: 271–5

This study looked at conventional repeat prescribing vs. pharmacist-managed prescribing. It concluded that pharmacist management was feasible. It identifies problems not always seen by GPs (in terms of compliance, adverse drug reactions or interactions), and could make savings (up to 18%) in the drug bill, i.e. it would outweigh the cost of the pharmacist.

Randomised controlled trial of clinical medication review by a pharmacist of elderly patients receiving repeat prescriptions in general practice
BMJ **2001; 323: 1340–3**

This trial concluded that a clinical pharmacist can conduct effective consultations with elderly patients in general practice to review their drugs. These reviews resulted in changes in patients' drugs and saved more than the cost of the intervention, without affecting the workload of GPs.

The British Lifestyle Survey 2001 (conducted by consumer researcher Mintel) found that the number of people who asked the pharmacist for advice had increased by 25%. Over-the-counter analgesic sales have risen by 41% and sales for remedies for coughs and colds have increased by 10%, all over the last 10 years.

Patient group directives

These are written instructions for the supply and administration of medicines by professionals other than doctors (e.g. pharmacists, nurses, health visitors). Their development came about following changes to the Medicines Act in 2000, the overall aim being to improve patient care. They are a recognised necessity with the advances in nurse prescribing. The process of drawing up a patient group directive (PGD) can be time-consuming, needs to be well thought out and involves a multidisciplinary team. For example, not only do pharmacists issuing emergency contraception need to be competent in assessing need and explaining related issues, but there needs to be a system for effective reimbursement for cost of the drug.

The PGD needs to be detailed, and once it is written it must be reviewed by at least one professional advisory group prior to circulation to practices. As with any published document it should be dated and have a plan for review.

Each directive must include the following:

- the name of the business to which it applies

- the date it comes into force and is due to expire

- a description of the medicines to which it applies

- the class of health professional who may supply or administer the medicine

- the signature of the doctor, dentist or pharmacist and appropriate health organisation

- the clinical condition to which it applies

- patients to be excluded
- when further advice should be sought.

Personal medical services

Personal medical services (PMS) is an alternative to GMS. The NHS Plan expected 30% of GPs to move to PMS by 2002 and all single-handers by 2004. This expectation was to change with the launch of the new GMS contract, which was to encompass some aspects of PMS.

PMS was actually introduced by the Conservative Government in the Primary Care Act 1997 after the initial concept had been introduced in *Choices and Opportunities*, a White Paper. It went live in April 1998 with a core contract that doctors had to fulfil. The contract was scrapped in favour of a broad framework with outcomes and targets to be agreed locally. Around 40% of GPs are working to PMS contracts.

The intention of PMS is to address local service issues and pilot new ways of delivering and improving services by allowing local flexibility. The emphasis is on local funding for local issues, which will hopefully attract GPs into areas with recruitment problems.

PMS covers what people would normally expect from GMS, but delivery can be different. The focus is on competitive services, achieving targets and a minimum of three audits per year. PMS providers will be accountable for delivery of National Service Frameworks and other key national clinical governance requirements (risk management, audits, workforce planning, etc.).

An Introduction to PMS is a GPC publication which covers the aims of PMS:

- promoting consistently high-quality services

- providing opportunities and incentives for primary care professionals to use their skills to the full

- providing more flexible employment opportunities

- addressing recruitment and retention problems

- reducing the bureaucracy involved in the management of primary care provision.

As would be expected, PMS has had a variable reception. As happens with all new developments, the initial money available (especially for growth) was quite substantial, but this is no longer the case. Also, interestingly, the PMS core contract for third-wavers is much more directive.

The King's Fund study entitled *Current thoughts on PMS so far* was published in October 2001. It concluded that PMS had so far been 'disappointing'.

Personal Medical Services Pilots: modernising primary care? states 'there is little strong or consistent evidence of a "PMS effect" on quality'.

A PMS contract is not enforceable by law, but both parties are subject to binding arbitration by the Secretary of State for Health.

Benefits of PMS

- It is locally negotiated so can reflect local circumstances.

- There was less management bureaucracy at the time it was launched.

- It enables flexible employment opportunities, with opportunities and incentives to develop skills.

- There is improved integration of primary healthcare teams.

- There are more services available for patients.
- It addresses some recruitment and retention problems in general practice.
- It promotes consistently high-quality services.
- It is practice based, not a contract with an individual doctor (i.e. illness, maternity leave, etc.), much like the new GMS contract.

PMS practices have the right to alter the quality and outcome frameworks if agreed with the primary care trust.

Drawbacks of PMS

- It is local not national, so is not aligned with national pay reviews.
- There is no agreement on pensions.
- There is annual renegotiation of the contract and this is then fixed for a year, which may compromise income.
- The local medical committee statutory levy is not automatically taken.
- Funding for growth reduced with each new wave.
- Discrepancies in earnings (where there is significantly more income than in GMS) are being looked into (i.e. to determine if there is provision of a better service for patients).

The new GMS contract: *Your Contract, Your Future*

www.bma.org.uk and www.doh.gov.uk

The Red Book – our terms of service – was renegotiated and costed, looking at the workload, infrastructure, practice expenses and skill-mix changes that were necessary.

The contract is between the primary care trust and the practice (i.e. there will be no individual lists) and will be for essential and additional services. The contract will safeguard premises, allowing for improvement and development in the interest of quality patient care. The final version was launched in April 2004.

Investing in general practice: the new GMS contract

The basis of the new GMS contract has been accepted and should:

- provide new mechanisms to allow practices greater flexibility to determine the range of services they wish to provide
- reward practices for delivering clinical and organisational quality and for improving the patient experience
- facilitate the modernisation of practice infrastructure, including premises and IT

- provide for unprecedented and guaranteed levels of investment through a gross investment guarantee

- support the delivery of a wider range of higher-quality services and empower patients to make the best use of primary care services

- simplify the regulatory regime.

UK expenditure on primary care should rise from £6.1 billion to £8 billion over 3 years (a 31% increase). One of the funding issues is that, as GPs, we have surprised politicians with our achievements in enhanced services, leading to anticipated shortfalls in budget allowances.

More flexible provision of services

All GMS practices will provide essential services and a range of enhanced services. Practices will have the opportunity to increase their income through opting to provide a wider range of enhanced services.

Primary care trusts are responsible for ensuring patient access is not compromised and by 31 December 2004 should have taken full responsibility for out-of-hours (6.30pm–8am weekdays, all weekends, bank holidays and public holidays) services. This will include GP co-operatives, NHS Direct/24, walk-in centres, paramedics, pharmacists, GP services in Accident and Emergency, commercial deputising services and social work services.

How will the money flow?

1 *Protected global sum*: paid directly to the practice from the primary care trust for essential and additional services. This represent a lot of the past Red Book payments.

2 *Enhanced services payments*: from the primary care trust; includes development money.

3 *Wisdom and experience payments*: from the primary care trust, for more senior doctors.

4 *Quality and outcome payments*:
   - infrastructure, e.g. premises, IT, staff
   - ten chronic disease frameworks and organisational achievements
   - aspiration – declared by the practice at the beginning of the year
   - reward – paid at the end of the year if aspirations are met.

Categorisation of services

Essential services

These are provided by every practice, and the service is initiated by the patient. They include the following:

- management of patients who are ill:
  - relevant health promotion
  - appropriate referral
- general management of patients who are terminally ill:
  - chronic disease management.

Additional services

Most practices would be expected to provide these, but could opt out if necessary (e.g. because of staff shortages):

- cervical screening
- contraceptive services
- vaccinations and immunisations
- child health surveillance
- maternity services (intrapartum care would be an enhanced service)
- minor surgery.

Enhanced services

These are essential or additional services delivered to a higher specific standard, as well as innovative services. They will allow primary care trusts to invest in areas such as routine home visits, patient transport, services for violent patients, etc.
   There will be:

- national direction with specifications and benchmark pricing which all primary care trusts must commission
- national minimum specifications and benchmark pricing that are not directed
- locally developed services.

Breadth of care will be rewarded through holistic care payments. This categorisation would allow GPs to:

- control their workload
- receive guaranteed resources
- opt out of additional services if they are unable to provide them
- offer innovative services.

New services will only ever be introduced when the necessary additional resources have been provided.

Rewarding quality and outcomes

The quality framework started with four main components, focusing on four domains each with key indicators.

1 *Clinical standards (10 areas)*: coronary heart disease, stroke or transient ischaemic attack, hypertension, diabetes, chronic obstructive airways disease, epilepsy, cancer, mental health, hypothyroidism and asthma.

2 *Organisational standards (5 areas)*: records and information about patients, information for patients, education and training, medicines management, and clinical and practice management.

3 *Experience of patients (2 areas)*: covering the services provided, how they are provided and their involvement in service development plans; this will involve a satisfaction survey and the consultation length offered.

4 *Additional services (4 areas)*: cervical screening, child health surveillance, maternity services and contraceptive services.

At the beginning of the year the practice receives a proportion of the quality payment for the standard aspired – the *aspiration payment*. Once the standard has been achieved, the practice receives the remainder – the *achievement payment*. There is also (in the first 3 years only) a *preparation payment*.

Exception reporting will be in place to ensure practices don't lose payment as a result of factors outside their control. Similarly, certain categories of patients will be excluded (e.g. those who are terminally ill, those on maximum medication, newly diagnosed patients, etc.).

As part of this original document, global sum payments were to be calculated on the Carr–Hill allocation formula. There were problems with the weighting of this, especially for practices with accurate practice lists. The allocation formula for the global sum will now be applied to the registered practice population from 1 April 2004. As a result of this and concerns over income a *minimum practice income guarantee* (MPIG) for the first few years has been confirmed.

After the first successful year the quality indicators are being reviewed and various panels have submitted their recommendations, including NICE. At the time of writing, nothing has been finalised. In light of the soon-to-be-published White Paper *Choosing Health*, there is a likelihood of an overall shift towards public health issues such as obesity.

A fresh new contract for GPs
BMJ 2002; 324: 1048–9

This is a firm critique of some of the philosophy behind the contract proposal. 'Currently allocation of resources only poorly reflects patients' needs. It focuses on individual GPs and fails to recognise the role of the practice team. Quality measures are sparse and crudely applied and perverse incentives often serve to reward poor quality services.' National pricing of the new contract (announced 19 April 2002) will take into account changing demands on primary care through an annual assessment of workload. If workload rises, new resources will be made available. In the future, GPs will be better able to control their workload. Incentives for GPs will change, i.e. more focus on quality.

NHS Cancer Plan

www.doh.gov.uk

This was introduced in September 2000 following a series of cancer guidelines, the aim being to improve cancer care and outcome in the NHS. The plan was developed by a multidisciplinary team, but for it to have any impact it will need 'local leadership and support'. Each primary care trust will have a cancer lead.

The Government will play its part by investing in the workforce and tackling shortages. There will be 1,000 new cancer specialists, and histopathology and radiography will also be targeted.

It is hoped that the plan will be achieved by increasing capacity through new ways of working and developing opportunities, as well as by education, recruitment and retention planning. Needless to say, a variety of opinions have been expressed in editorials and in the letters pages, ranging from 'excellent, simple, clear, GP and patient centred' to 'a waste of money, politically motivated and barely enough investment to keep up with the increasing incidence of cancer'.

The plan has four main aims:

1 to save more lives

2 to ensure that people with cancer get professional support and care, as well as the best treatment

3 to tackle inequalities in health that mean unskilled workers are twice as likely to die from cancer as professionals

4 to build a future through cancer research and preparation for a genetic revolution.

There are three new commitments:

1 to reduce smoking in manual workers from 32% (in 1998) to 26% by 2010

2 to reduce waiting times for diagnosis and treatment to 1 month (from an urgent cancer referral to starting treatment) by 2005

3 to invest an extra £50 million in hospices and specialist palliative care.

Also discussed is the role of promoting a healthier diet, the five-a-day programme. As well as raising public awareness, children aged 4–6 years will be able to have a piece of fruit every day if they want (currently this works with fruit being offered at school instead of dessert and tuck, and having dedicated fruit tuck days where fruit is the only option).

There are plans to extend cancer screening in the following ways.

- *Breast cancer screening*: this will be extended to women aged 65–70 years by 2004, and will be available on request to those over 70 years of age.

- *Cervical screening*: the programme will be upgraded and unnecessary repeats reduced.

- *Colorectal cancer*: pilots have now been completed and are currently under discussion.

- *Prostate cancer*: prostate specific antigen (PSA) tests will be available to empower men to make their own choices. No formal programme is planned, as too many questions remain unanswered.

- *Ovarian cancer*: screening trials are in progress.

Finally, there will be investment in research, in particular the National Cancer Research Institute. Advances in genetics will lead to a greater understanding of inherited susceptibility in the future. As things stand, the cancer genetics service needs a strategic framework to develop further. The Harper Report recommended that primary care should be the principal focus for clinical cancer genetics. This in turn came from the Calman–Hine Report, which recommended that there should be networks of cancer care in research, assessment, diagnosis and treatment.

National Institute for Clinical Excellence

www.nice.org.uk

NICE was launched in England and Wales in 1999 and aims to produce guidance in three areas of health:

1 *health technologies* – both new and existing, including drugs, treatments and procedures

2 *clinical practice* – appropriate treatment and care of people with specific diseases and conditions

3 *public health* – promotion of good health and prevention of ill health.

It was created to produce guidelines for health professionals and must ensure its advice is based on rigorous analysis of all the available evidence, both clinical and economic. It also seeks advice on social, ethical and moral questions from the citizens' council, a team of individuals representative of the population of England and Wales. Its decisions are advisory, not mandatory, but local health organisations are obliged to review their management against guidelines as they are published. There is a requirement to provide funding within 3 months for medicines and technologies recommended by NICE.

As part of NICE there is a Referral Practice Project Steering Group, which is responsible for the recently published guidelines.

Following the controversial reversal of its decision on Zanamivir, since April 2001 all evidence has to be open. However, there are still concerns that NICE may be influenced by industry or patient organisations.

Wrong SIGN, NICE mess: is national guidance distorting allocation of resources?
BMJ 2001; 323: 743–5

This article discusses the Scottish Intercollegiate Guidelines Network (SIGN) and NICE. The authors state that the way forward to remedy some of the problems is for NICE to become a recognised rationing agency. It should say no to relatively costly and ineffective new drugs. The authors suggest implementing a fixed-growth budget for new technologies, distributed to primary care trusts.

The failings of NICE
BMJ 2000; 321: 1363 (Editorial)

This editorial was written in the early days, criticising NICE (and politicians) for not admitting to its role of rationing within the NHS.

From guidance to practice: why NICE is not enough
BMJ 2002; 324: 842–5

This article considers that NICE will work if the health service supports and implements the changes that it promotes. At present this is not the case.

There are some questions in the exam that may ask you to consider the differences between implicit and explicit rationing. It is thought that NICE will encourage implicit rationing by delay (waiting lists, discrimination among the elderly and the mentally ill) and dilution (of specialist care, e.g. two nurses instead of four on an elderly care ward to cover the drug costs). This was part of the reason that the authors of 'NICE mess' cited above felt that NICE should also be able to refuse to give guidance on some areas if it felt it was not appropriate to do so.

The House of Commons Health Committee has conducted an enquiry into NICE (January 2002). This considered to what extent the institute has provided independent, clear and credible guidance, and also whether it has enabled patients to have quicker access to drugs known to be effective, and whether guidance is accepted locally and acted upon. The Health Select Committee and the Consumers' Association have criticised the work of NICE as flaws have been found in guidance issued.

Many independent authors consider that it is only a matter of time before NICE guidance becomes mandatory, and they continue to discuss the serious concerns as to how statistical tools are decided upon and the ultimate conclusions reached.

One of the most significant human rights issues is that NICE has released a statement that in the future it will recommend against treating patients for smoking-related conditions if they continue to smoke. Its current thought is that age and lifestyle factors that may have caused disease shouldn't influence guidance on the use of interventions unless they are likely to compromise the effectiveness of the intervention.

National Service Frameworks

National Service Frameworks (NSFs) were proposed in the 1998 White Paper *A First Class Service: quality in the new NHS* as part of the Government's agenda to drive up quality and reduce unacceptable variations in health and social services across the UK. They have been proposed as accompaniments to NICE and identified as priorities in *Modernising Health and Social Services: national priorities guidance for 1999/ 2000–2000/01*.

The standards will be set by NICE and NSFs, delivered by clinical governance, and underpinned by self-regulation and lifelong learning. The Healthcare Commission, the National Performance Assessment Framework and the National Survey of Patients will be used to monitor the NSFs. Performance will be assessed through a small number of national milestones and high-level performance indicators.

There will be advances and changes during the implementation of the NSFs. Therefore they will have to evolve if they are to stay relevant and credible in such a changing environment. Similarly, the need for learning and development (organisational, professional and personal) is recognised.

Objectives of NSFs

These are as follows:

1 to address problems that affect quality of NHS care

2 to tackle variations in:
- agreed standards of care
- data collection and audit
- local provision of national services
- funding and resources
- involvement with non-NHS agencies.

Appraisal

www.appraisals.nhs.uk

Appraisal is a formative and developmental process. It is about identifying developmental needs as part of a personal development plan, for example, and at the time of writing does not have a performance management role. It is a yearly requirement that was introduced in April 2002.

You can register for, and access, the appraisal toolkit by logging on to the above website. You can then complete your appraisal for your appraiser online.

GP experiences of partner and extended peer appraisal: a qualitative study
Br J Gen Pract 2005; 55: 539–43

This paper explored different views to approaches that could be adopted for appraisal. A total of 66 GPs took part in the study (46 had a partner appraisal and 20 an external appraiser). This was followed up after 6 months by a questionnaire, and 13 GPs were interviewed in depth. It was felt that clarification in the role of appraisal and revalidation was needed. Given the potentially charged nature of appraisal, there was a risk of collusion between appraiser and appraisee, which may lead to a superficial appraisal.

Personal development plans

The need for personal development plans (PDPs) has been recognised and evolved from the shortcomings of 30 hours of undirected Postgraduate Educational Allowance (PGEA), as well as media attention that has focused on recent medical scandals (e.g. the Bristol Inquiry and the Shipman case). Revalidation will require us to demonstrate our learning, which we will have to map out according to our own individual needs. These will in turn be determined by priorities that are dictated by the influences around us, such as national expectations, primary care groups, and practice and personal needs.

Good Medical Practice in General Practice, published by the Royal College of General Practitioners, states that an excellent GP:

- is up to date and regularly reviews their knowledge
- uses these reviews to develop practice and their personal development plan
- uses a range of methods to monitor and meet their educational needs.

A First Class Service: quality in the new NHS is a 1998 Government publication which states that lifelong learning will give NHS staff the knowledge necessary to offer the most effective and high-quality care to patients. Continuous professional development (CPD) programmes need to meet the learning needs of the individual, inspire public confidence in their skills and also meet the wider developmental needs of the NHS.

The NHS Plan, published in July 2000, is about staff working smarter not harder. All doctors employed within the NHS have been required to participate in annual appraisals and clinical audit since 2001.

The advantages of personal development plans can be summarised as follows:

- personal satisfaction
- personally relevant
- more flexible than the PGEA system
- aspirations are achieved
- helps personal reflection
- fulfils contract requirements
- improved patient care
- more cost-effective.

The disadvantages can be summarised as follows:

- can lead to isolation
- loss of objectivity
- may be overwhelming
- needs a support network or mentor
- needs more time investment than PGEA
- can be seen as time-wasting and unnecessary by self-motivating learners
- may be reinforcing skills that are already adequate.

Writing a PDP/practice development plan

In addition to a PDP, when working in a GP setting/partnership, there will be a requirement for a practice development plan. This is based on the same principles as a PDP.

Identifying learning needs

These represent the gap between the way things are now and the way they should be or how you want them to be in the future. Learning needs can be identified by keeping lists, reviewing referrals, conducting audits, significant event analysis, asking colleagues, i.e. 360 degree appraisal, etc. (known as the 'Johari window').

Setting learning objectives

Objectives may involve knowledge, skills, attitude, etc. Success can be looked at by reflection, feedback, audit, reduction in demand, etc.

Identifying resource implications and timescales

This means that plans should be achievable.

Seeking evidence of achievement

A formal PDP is one stage of a continuous process. The evidence can be used to make a learning portfolio (i.e. a long-term record of past experience and future aspirations) containing workload logs, case descriptions, videos, audits, patient surveys, reflection, significant event analysis, etc. This is the 'cradle to grave' idea.

Although the plan has now been formalised, conscientious doctors have been doing this for years, as it is the fundamental principle that underpins adult learning, educational theories and learning cycles. We all want to develop and work within an effective team, improve clinical care, plan constructively and provide mechanisms of accountability. PDPs are a starting point for this, which will also help us bid for resources in the future.

Revalidation: professional self-regulation

www.revalidationuk.info and www.appraisaluk.info

Revalidation will be an episodic process to demonstrate fitness to practise to the professional regulator (the General Medical Council). The fifth report of the Shipman Inquiry provided a thorough analysis of a doctor's fitness to practise. Partly because of the negative media attention attracted by recent cases such as the Bristol Inquiry and the Shipman Inquiry, the GMC is undergoing a period of reform aimed mainly at proving that it is capable of regulating the profession. However, the responsibility for basic competence is that of the individual doctor – it always has been and always will be. There will always be other factors that allow incompetence and poorly performing professionals to be brought to our attention (e.g. prescribing data, complaints, new contract fulfilment, referral types – not specifically quantity but quality, etc.). One of the difficulties highlighted by various editorials is how to make revalidation stimulating and worthwhile for the majority of doctors, while at the same time sensitive enough to pick out those who are performing poorly.

Revalidation for Clinical General Practice was produced by a revalidation party for the Royal College of General Practitioners. It anticipates that revalidation will be related to a number of different systems, e.g. clinical governance, accredited professional development, appraisal, GMC performance procedures, etc.

The criteria they have identified for revalidation to work are as follows.

- It should be understood by the public and be credible.
- It should identify unacceptable performance.
- It should identify good performance.
- It should be supported by the profession and support the profession.
- It should be practical and feasible.
- It should not put any GPs or practices at an advantage or disadvantage.

Revalidation should be a continuous summative process with episodic submission and assessment of fitness to practise, having been through an annual appraisal process. Evidence should be drawn from the doctor's day-to-day practice.

The original proposed layout for the folder is as follows.

- Section 1: Personal registration details, also providing a contact address.
- Section 2: What you do – information about your field of practice, actual activities and time spent each week.
- Section 3: Information about your practice, including the following:
  - audit and results
  - critical incidents: your role and changes made
  - structured reviews and surveys of your practice by other professionals
  - routine indicators: PACT data, admissions, etc.

- investigations by, e.g. RCGP, National Clinical Assessment Service, and their results
- details of articles and books published, also qualifications gained
- subscriptions to professional journals
- your role in producing guidelines and protocols
- complaints and resulting changes
- training and teaching roles
- detail your own health problems or convictions
- disciplinary action by an employer
- confirm you have not knowingly left out any relevant information.

Where are we with revalidation?

The initial basis of revalidation plans is discussed above. In April 2003, the GMC changed the plans in the following ways.

- The proposal to evaluate doctors by revalidation panels was dropped.

- Doctors who work in quality-assured environments where clinical governance operates, and who have annual appraisals, could use their appraisal as their application for revalidation.

- Doctors who work outside the NHS have to collect documents as described above (i.e. a two-tier system).

- Following concerns by Dame Janet Smith (in the Shipman report), a clinical governance certificate, signed by the employing organisation, also needs to be submitted.

There are several reasons why revalidation has been postponed. The Chief Medical Officer is conducting an enquiry into the GMC's role following concerns raised by the fifth Shipman report. It is thought that initial changes may have been brought about because of the cost of revalidating 30,000 doctors a year and the duplication of current systems with little evidence that it would stop another Shipman.

GMC and the future of revalidation. Failure to act on good intentions
BMJ 2005; 330: 1144–7 (Education and Debate)

This article was written by Aneez Esmail (professor in general practice) with a following commentary by Mayur Lakhani (a member of the council). It discusses some of the issues above and gives a good narrative into the history, problems and ways forward for revalidation.

GMC and the future of revalidation: a way forward
BMJ 2005; 330: 1326–8

This article by Mayur Lakhani outlines ten guiding principles for revalidation. It includes the recognition that revalidation is summative, needs clear criteria, needs lay involvement, must be in addition to appraisal and clinical governance, and should include local certification. It also advocates that the reliability of information should be ensured, there should be alternative routes for revalidation, a tighter definition of a managed clinical environment and that the standards should be consistent across the whole medical profession (where possible).

Clinical governance

www.cgsupport.org (clinical governance support website)

Where revalidation is a professional-based measure to ensure high standards of care, clinical governance has more of a management base, being accountable to the Government through the primary care trusts. Its aim is to improve the quality of services offered in the NHS and safeguard high standards, as well as to create an environment in which clinical excellence will flourish.

It was published in a Labour Government White Paper to highlight to the public that the NHS will not tolerate anything less than the best. This is to be achieved in a no-blame, questioning, learning culture.

In 1999, an NHS Clinical Governance Support Team was established to support the development and implementation of clinical governance. This team is now part of the Modernisation Agency. NICE will develop guidelines for standards expected of general practitioners.

The Healthcare Commission (which consists of GPs, community nurses and lay people) is a PCT-based group. Its function is to look at clinical governance in practices and to try to effect necessary change. It will visit each PCT every 4 years and select practices at random. It can report directly to the Health Secretary if necessary.

The Government has done for medicine as it did for teaching and created *beacon practice* status for those most worthy. These practices demonstrate high standards in access, patient care, health improvement, etc. They are paid a nominal £4,000/year and in return are expected to promote their way of working, mainly through 12 open days per year at the practice for others to learn by example.

Each GP has a responsibility to provide a high quality of care and to audit this. Patients need to be confident that their doctor is up to date and offering effective treatment. Clinical governance is an effective tool for monitoring and improving quality of care in general practice.

The role of clinical governance as a strategy for quality improvement in primary care
Br J Gen Pract 2002; 52(Suppl.): S12–S17

This paper considers the process of implementing clinical governance in primary care and its impact on quality improvement. It states that success for implementation requires a multi-level approach to change (GP, PCT, NHS, etc.) and also that there are three overlapping sets of issues which enhance implementation, namely the environment (context), the leaders and the implementers or users of the change. The whole of this supplement looks at quality issues.

Improving the quality of care through clinical governance
BMJ 2001; 322: 1580–2

This is the third part of the series in the *BMJ*. One of the main obstacles envisaged in implementing a clinical governance team is the limited resources.

Making clinical governance work
BMJ 2005; 329: 679–82 (Education and Debate)

This discussion opens with the statement that clinical governance is 'by far the most high-profile vehicle for securing culture change in the new NHS'. The main points made are that:

- clinicians should be at the heart of clinical governance

- failing to take account of the scope of the clinician's work will result in their disengagement from management

- integrated care pathways are needed for common conditions

- healthcare professionals need support and systematic evaluation of their performance.

Primary care groups

PCGs were set up on 1 April 1999, working with patients and health authority representatives to develop healthcare needs in local communities following the Government's White Paper *The New NHS: modern, dependable*.
   The aim was that PCGs would ultimately develop trust status and take over from the health authority.
   There were four levels of PCG, depending on responsibility.

- Level 1 – supports the health authority in commissioning.

- Level 2 – develops budget responsibility.

- Level 3 – free-standing body accountable to the health authority for commissioning (i.e. primary care trust).

- Level 4 – as for Level 3, but also covers provision of community services.

Primary care trusts

A PCT is run by its board and the PCT Professional Executive Committee (PEC). The board itself comprises three heads, who are responsible for strategic planning:

- the chief executive, usually an NHS manager

- the PCT chairman, a lay person appointed by the Appointments Commission

- the PEC chairman, usually a GP.

There is also a medical director (who is usually not on the board), who is responsible for the day-to-day running of the clinical services.

Practice-based commissioning

www.nhsalliance.org.uk

Implementing the Vision was a report in 2000 by the NHS Alliance that called for multi-level commissioning (the budget having been created in response to the recognised need in the NHS Plan). In 2002, the Alliance published *Refocusing Commissioning for Primary Care Trusts* and then in 2004, *Practice-led Commissioning – a no nonsense guide.* They have been very keen from the outset for practice-based commissioning (PBC) to be seen as distinct from fundholding, describing it in the following ways.

- It is based on partnerships at many levels, so it encourages teamwork (there is no personal gain to be made from savings) and reinvestment for the good of all.

- The proposal is a clinical vision about what we want to achieve for our patients by improving quality of services.

Practices are under no obligation to participate until December 2006, but when they do take on the role, they will be expected to manage the commissioning of services, budgets and an element of risk associated with this (although they would not be held directly responsible for any overspend). Around 40% of practices in England are involved in PBC and have started organising their preferred commissioning group (for which there remains little official guidance).

MedEconomics (April 2005) published a special edition on PBC, which is as useful, if not more so, than the NHS Alliance documentation. It drew up a 10-stage approach to PBC.

1 Find out all you can about it.

2 Discuss it with everybody.

3 Plan what you will commission.

4 Decide which services you will commission jointly.

5 Agree the budget with the PCT.

6 Sign on the dotted line.

7 Allow for patient choice.

8 Recoup your initial costs and management expenses.

9 Monitor your budget.

10 Use efficiency gains.

Dr Jenner (in *Doctor* January 2005) discusses the new guidance and how it has moved from original thoughts in the following areas.

- *Inevitability of PBC* – there are no targets, but by 2008 all practices will be involved in PBC.

- *Incentives for practices* – there will be no cap (previously 50%) on the amount of savings.

- *Accountability for practices* is to follow national priorities – national and local targets must be delivered (including Choose and Book, access, waiting list initiatives, etc.).

- *Single practice or locality commissioning* – the new guidance tips the balance in favour of locality groups (the King's Fund suggests that you need a patient population of 30,000 to manage a total healthcare budget over 3 years).

- *Budget setting* – budgets will be set at 2003/04 levels of referral (to avoid the initial increase seen in fundholding, where referrals were boosted in the first year to increase budgets) and then move to a shared formula.

- *Risk management* – practices are not financially responsible for overspends, that lies with the PCT, which can intervene if it is thought the commissioning group will be overspent.

- *Arbitration* – the SHA can convene a panel of two GPs, one practice manager and the PCT finance director to resolve issues.

Medical error

To err is human. Individual mistakes are inevitable, but complacency will always be unacceptable.

Reducing medical mishaps is fundamental to improving quality. 'First do no harm' is part of our Hippocratic oath. Harm is done every day and it needs skill to translate these negative events into useful information. For this to happen there needs to be some type of reporting to enable system changes which will improve patient safety.

Doctors tend to overestimate their ability to function flawlessly under adverse conditions such as fatigue, time pressure and high anxiety. Aviation and other non-medical, 'hands-on' industries have developed incident reporting where the focus is on *near misses*. There are incentives for voluntary reporting, confidentiality is ensured and the emphasis is on data collection, analysis and improvement, rather than a punitive approach.

Gaps in continuity of care that lead to near misses or harm can be described at three levels: individual people, stages or processes. Increasing safety can be achieved by understanding and reinforcing our ability to bridge these gaps. Despite all the defences, barriers and safeguards that are inbuilt, mistakes will continue to happen, so the aim should be to minimise the risks at each stage.

For example, system changes that would improve patient safety would include:

- reducing complexity and having a systematic approach

- optimising information processing with awareness of workload

- automating wisely (i.e. use IT to support human operation rather than because it is available)

- using constraints to restrict certain actions, and double-checking critical processes

- mitigating the unwanted side effects of change (e.g. test on a small scale to try to predict problems and monitor the outcome)

- training in safety issues for all staff

- regular audit.

Examples of where this approach has been successful are seen in the pharmaceutical industry, with drugs and anaesthetic attachments.

Almost an entire issue of the *British Medical Journal* (18 March 2000) was dedicated to medical error. The 'error prevention movement' has accelerated, and major changes are occurring in the way that we think about and carry out our daily work. There is an undercurrent of more slowly evolving cultural change in our learning, responsibilities and ability to admit fallibility.

For risk assessment (i.e. reporting of near misses) to be successful, incidents need to be analysed in an organisational way, rather than on a personal basis. Formal protocols need to be developed to ensure systematic, comprehensive and efficient investigations. As always, training needs to be part of the developing programme if it is to be a standardised and effective tool.

Acknowledgement of 'no fault' medical injury: review of patients' hospital records in New Zealand
BMJ 2003; 326: 79–80

This review reported that doctors in counties with a no fault compensation system for medical injuries were more likely to report mistakes.

Should systems reporting be voluntary?

An example of voluntary reporting is the Safe Medical Devices Act 1990. Reporting is fundamental to the broad goal of error reduction. *Non-punitive, confidential, voluntary* reporting programmes provide more useful information about errors and their causes than mandatory reporting, for the following reasons.

- There is no fear of retribution.

- The depth of information is the key to understanding the problem. If reporting is forced, then the primary motivation is self-protection and adherence to requirement, not to help others avoid making the same mistake.

In the *BMJ* issue referred to above (18 March 2000), a number of papers and editorials highlighted the need to move away from individual blame towards an organisational approach where we acknowledge that mistakes are inevitable. By doing this, we could build systems to prevent such mistakes occurring and have a means of identifying them early (i.e. moving away from the *personal approach* towards a *systems approach*).

However, as things change in the future in the name of *continuous quality improvement*, it must be remembered that the person who makes the mistake needs help too – a point that is all too easy to forget and often overlooked.

Learning from adverse incidents involving medical devices
BMJ 2002; 325: 272–5

The NHS is perceived to have a poor record of learning from incidents, despite the efforts of the Medical Devices Agency to issue safety warnings. This study found that adverse incidents were typically caused by alignment of different factors, but that good practice can prevent errors becoming incidents.

The World Alliance for Patient Safety

At the launch of the World Alliance in Washington in October 2004, the WHO and its key partners announced a series of important actions intended to reduce harm caused to patients. These included the following.

- The global patient safety challenge – focusing on healthcare-associated infection.

- Patients for patient safety – involving patient organisations in Alliance work.

- Taxonomy for patient safety – ensuring consistency of concepts, principles and terminologies.

- Research for patient safety – promoting existing interventions and co-ordinating international efforts to develop solutions.

- Reporting and learning – generating best-practice guidelines for existing and new reporting systems.

The National Reporting and Learning System (NRLS) for adverse events and near misses was launched alongside the Alliance's report to encourage healthcare professionals to report incidents on a confidential basis.

Medication and safety

Building a Safer NHS for Patients: improving medication safety was launched in February 2004. It is a paper that looks at causes and frequency of medication errors and sets out a framework for a common quality of care throughout the NHS (taking further steps to achieve the aims of the Chief Medical Officer's Report, *An Organisation with a Memory*). It estimates that potentially serious errors occur in between 1 in 1,000 and 1 in 10,000 scripts, most of which are identified before any harm is done. The report considers medication processes generally, high-risk patient groups, high-risk drugs and organisational changes.

The Medicines Commission and the Committee on the Safety of Medicines are to be replaced by the Commission on Human Medicines, which will:

- advise ministers on licensing policies

- have overall responsibility for drug safety issues

- advise on appointment of other professional bodies serving the Medicines and Healthcare Products Regulatory Agency

- hear initial appeals from drug companies when a licence has been rejected.

National Clinical Assessment Service

This was established in April 2001 as part of the Government's commitment to quality. Its purpose is to investigate and assist doctors, if necessary, to resolve problems in performance at an early stage when they have been unable to resolve them at a local level. Such doctors are referred to the National Clinical Assessment Service by their employers or by themselves, *not* by patients.

There may be some overlap with the Healthcare Commission.

Assessments are all confidential, the only exception being where a statutory power (e.g. the police or the GMC) requires information.

National Patient Safety Agency

www.npsa.nhs.uk/rcatoolkit

The role of the National Patient Safety Agency (NPSA) is to promote an open and fair reporting culture, collecting, collating, categorising and coding adverse incidents, looking for patterns and trends, and acting on identified risks.

The NPSA was established in July 2001 to improve patient safety by running a national reporting system to log adverse clinical events and near misses, so that lessons can be shared and learned from in a blame-free way.

GPs have to report all incidents where a patient was, or could have been, seriously harmed. This follows the publication of a document entitled *A Commitment to Quality, a Quest for Excellence* in June 2001.

The NPSA document *Doing Less Harm* applies the reporting rule to all incidents, including anaphylaxis and unexpected death in the surgery (both of which are categorised as 'red'). Other incidents will be categorised as green, yellow or orange, depending on their severity.

In 2005, the NPSA introduced the *Being Open Policy*, a further document encouraging healthcare professionals to be frank about their mistakes. This will be introduced to all NHS organisations by June 2006. There are three main issues to this policy.

1 The principle is that when something goes wrong you should be open, apologise, investigate, learn and provide support.

2 Patient safety investigations are disclosable if a court case results, but the benefits of being open could outweigh the costs.

3 There should be exemption from disciplinary action when reporting incidents with a view to improving patient safety.

Healthcare Commission

This is a body representing the Government, which is made up of GPs, nurses and lay people, who look at clinical governance at a primary care group (PCG) level every 4 years. They can report underperforming PCGs to the Health Secretary. They will mainly investigate organisational systems.

New proposals are being suggested in the NHS Reform and Health Care Professions bill where the Healthcare Commission will be able to recommend that the Health Secretary takes 'special measures' against failing GP practices. This new bill will also create an office within the Healthcare Commission to collect and publish statistics on primary care services and give patient groups the right to inspect all GP premises.

Significant event analysis

This process is known by various names, including significant event audit, critical event audit or analysis, and significant event review. It can include examples of when things go right as well as wrong. It can be clinical or non-clinical and it can involve anyone in the team, the point being that such events are powerful motivators for change, and the questions that may be raised could identify a previously unidentified learning need. Significant event analysis should be felt to be a positive experience by all those involved.

How can significant event analysis be organised?

- Decide who is to be involved (e.g. doctors, nurses, receptionists, administration/ office staff).

- How are they to be organised (e.g. regular meetings, triggered by specific cases)?

- The time interval after the event should not be too long, otherwise momentum is lost and details are forgotten. This is especially important if new ideas are to be implemented.

- The meeting should be free of interruptions.

- A suitable environment is needed. Sometimes it is beneficial to be outside the workplace.

- Set ground rules (e.g. confidentiality and anonymity).

- Appoint a chairperson and a scribe for appropriate record keeping.

- The agenda may include the following points:
  - Why has the significant event been chosen?
  - What do people want to achieve by analysing it?
  - What are the facts of the case? These are often circulated before the meeting.
  - What issues are raised (e.g. care, communication)?
  - What went well?
  - What went badly and how can things be improved? (Shortcomings and things that are amenable to change should be highlighted. But avoid personal attacks and keep comments constructive.)
  - What actions should be taken?
    - (i)   Formulate a plan.
    - (ii) Prioritise points.
    - (iii) Decide on a timescale.
    - (iv) Consider how success can be determined.

Medical/clinical audit

Audit definitions have evolved somewhat from Maurin's 1976 thoughts (in terms of it being a general counting exercise) to the modern-day Government's definition in *Working for Patients*, which defines audit as 'the systematic critical analysis of the quality of medical care, including procedures used for the diagnosis and treatment, the use of resources and the resulting outcome and quality of life for the patients' (i.e. it is a much more active approach).

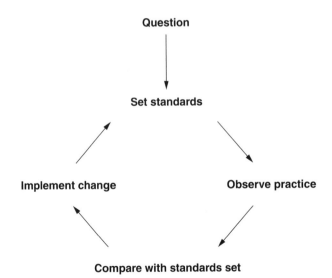

Summary of the audit cycle.

Donabedian (1982) identified three major categories:

1 audit of *structure* – delivery of care (e.g. appointments)

2 audit of *process* – how patients are treated (e.g. looking at prescriptions)

3 audit of *outcome* – what ultimately happens (e.g. mortality, morbidity).

In *Duties of a Doctor*, the GMC describes audit as an essential professional responsibility. The Royal College of General Practitioners Information Service (No.17) published an information leaflet on medical audit in March 2001 (www.rcgp.org.uk).
    Audit is a means by which we can look systematically and critically at our work – it is the final stage of evidence-based medicine. It is not research (research is done to find out what best practice is). Audit is a measure of performance against a predetermined standard. It can highlight problems, encourage change, reduce errors and demonstrate good care.
    Audit is increasingly part of clinical governance and will become an integral part of revalidation. Help with audits can be found in primary care audit groups and medical audit advisory groups.

Complaints

A complaint is an expression of dissatisfaction that requires a response. The number of complaints against GPs has doubled in the past 10 years. Handling complaints well puts things right for the individual who has received a poor service, and it allows those services to be improved. Resolving complaints at an early stage is the ultimate aim.
    The main complaints encountered in general practice are as follows:

• delayed diagnosis or failure to make a diagnosis, or an incorrect diagnosis

• failure to visit

• surgery appointment times/availability

• staff attitudes/rudeness

• inadequate examination

• refusal to refer.

If an individual wishes to make a complaint, this should be done within 6 months of the incident, or from finding out that there was something to complain about. The general consensus is that a complaint should be made within 1 year.
    The *NHS complaints procedure* has three stages:

1 local resolution (with or without an independent lay conciliator liaising between the two parties)

2 a convenor, who can request an independent review or refer back for local resolution

3 the Ombudsman (Health Service Commissioner).

Complaints procedure in primary care

Following the publication of the Wilson Report, *Being Heard*, in 1994, the complaints procedure was revised in 1996 and is in the process of being updated again, following the publication of a response document, *Reforming the NHS Complaints Procedure: a listening document* (which can be downloaded from www.doh.gov.uk). The GMC has published several booklets that explain the complaints procedure and how to raise concerns.

All practices should have a written and publicised complaints procedure explaining who patients should speak to and what to expect (required as part of our contract). In the event of a complaint:

1 the nominated person or deputy should interview the complainant and again explain the procedure

2 complaints must be acknowledged within 2 working days, or at the time if verbal

3 the complainant should receive a written response within 10 working days (20 if it is a hospital complaint). The response should:
   (i)   summarise the complaint
   (ii) explain the patient's view of the complaint
   (iii) apologise, if this is appropriate
   (iv) describe the outcome and steps taken
   (v)   explain the next step, how to contact the health authority/primary care trust if the complainant is still unhappy.

Ensure that if the complaint is made by someone other than the patient, consent is obtained from the patient. Be clear and concise, and try to avoid medical terminology. If you do have to use medical terms, explain them clearly.

Practices should:

• keep a separate complaints file

• include complaints statistics in the contract report, and for revalidation in the future

• hold practice meetings on complaints and how to manage them.

The NHS complaints procedure is not about tackling disciplinary action, which would need to be investigated by a professional disciplinary body after having been referred by the primary care trust to a disciplinary panel. Disciplinary measures can only be taken if a GP has failed to comply with their terms of service. Furthermore, the procedure does not deal with claims for financial compensation, private healthcare treatment or events about which an individual is already taking legal action.

The Independent Complaints Advocacy Service is the NHS body that will help patients or families who wish to lodge a complaint against the NHS.

Current issues

The Healthcare Commission is advocating a new complaints system which would allow underperforming GPs to be identified relatively quickly.
The main recommendations are:

- anonymous complaints to be logged

- patients to be given more say in the appointment of new partners

- improved patient information on what to expect from the doctor–patient relationship.

The other main point being reviewed is local resolution, in that patients have to complain to their practice and cannot choose to bypass this to avoid unpleasantness and the possibility of being struck off (i.e. the possibility of dysfunctional relationships developing).

Consent

The *Reference Guide to Consent for Examination or Treatment* is a 30-page document produced by the Department of Health's Good Practice in Consent Advisory Group, which summarises legal requirements and good practice requirements on consent. *The 12 Key Points on Consent: the law in England* is available at www.doh.gov.uk.
The document is relevant to all healthcare professionals, including students. It does not cover consent issues for the use of organs or tissues after death, nor does it include participation in observational studies or the use of personal information.
It is worth noting that the law changes depending on different test cases that are brought. Also the European Human Rights Act will probably have some effect on English law.
The BMA ethics department published the *Consent Tool Kit* booklet in March 2000, which is aimed at improving understanding and the practice of obtaining valid consent. Similarly, the GMC has published *Seeking Patient's Consent: the ethical considerations* and *Good Medical Practice*. The first covers the issues of consent, the second raises awareness of the importance of consent in everyday practice.
The approach taken to consent is fundamental to the doctor–patient relationship, and highlights an individual's ethical viewpoint on a patient's autonomy. Tony Hope wrote a helpful ethically based piece on consent in *Medicine* in October 2000. He suggests a quick three-point check on legal validity.

1 Is the patient properly informed?

2 Is the patient competent to give consent?

3 Did the patient give consent voluntarily (without coercion)?

From a legal point of view, consent provides the patient with a power of veto. Without consent, a patient could successfully sue a doctor for battery. Technically, touching another person without consent constitutes battery (i.e. the patient does not need to have suffered harm). Similarly, a doctor could be found negligent if they have not given the patient certain relevant information to allow that patient to give informed consent.

The fact that a person comes to see a doctor or is admitted to hospital does not imply consent to any examination, investigation or treatment. In giving/refusing consent it is important that the patient understands the reasons behind treatment, the associated risks and benefits, and the consequences if they refuse treatment (even the issuing of a prescription requires consent). It does not matter how the patient gives consent. It can be written, verbal or non-verbal. A signature does not prove consent is valid. Documentation of information given and consent is important.

The GMC is reviewing consent as part of the review of its core guidance document (*Good Medical Practice*), and NICE has similarly published guidance on consent issues. In UK law, the term 'informed consent' does not exist, explicit consent is required. Legal duties are defined by statute (e.g. the Children's Act 1989 and the Human Rights Act 1998) and by common law (which is general principles from specific cases). There is also guidance on the use of chaperones, which should be offered when any intimate (breast, genital or rectal) examination or procedure is to be carried out. Practices are advised to have a chaperone policy in place. This follows publication of the Ayling Report (2000) by the Department of Health.

Fraser guidelines

Confidentiality is important for all patients, but many young patients think that their parents can have access to their records, and that they have to be over 16 to see a health professional without their parents. This is not the case.

A young person can consent to treatment if:

- they understand the doctor's advice
- the doctor cannot persuade the young person to inform their parents, or allow the doctor to inform their parents, that they are seeking contraceptive advice
- they are very likely to begin, or continue having, intercourse with or without contraceptive treatment
- unless they receive contraceptive treatment, the young person's physical or mental health (or both) are likely to suffer.

Confidentiality

The success of the doctor–patient relationship is dependent on a number of factors. Confidentiality ('secrecy and discretion') has a therapeutically significant role, and has been fundamental to our code of practice since before the Hippocratic oath. Without its assurance, patients may be reluctant to give doctors the information they need in order to provide good care. Information that is learned about a patient belongs to that patient (even after death), and they have the right to determine who has access to it.

GMC Guidelines on Confidentiality: protecting and providing information

These provide information on confidentiality, holding and disclosing information. The new edition (2004) takes into account the Health and Social Care Act (2001) and is more flexible, because further changes are expected in laws around confidentiality. These guidelines do not have the force of law, but are taken seriously by the courts.

Disclosure to a third party, the Data Protection Act

A doctor's legal obligation of confidentiality is best seen as a public rather than a private interest (i.e. the obligation is not absolute, and in some situations the law allows or even obliges doctors to breach confidentiality). You are advised to discuss issues with your defence union if there is any ambiguity surrounding the need to disclose the information being requested.

Examples of circumstances where a doctor must breach confidentiality include termination of pregnancy (Abortion Act 1967), notifiable diseases (1984 Act), births and deaths (Births, Deaths and Registration Act 1953), and forms for incapacity benefit. The police can request names and addresses (but not clinical details) of persons alleged to be guilty under the Road Traffic Accident Act (1988).

Examples of circumstances where doctors have discretion to breach confidentiality include imparting information to other members of the healthcare team, a patient driving who is not fit to drive (the GMC advises informing the DVLA) and where a third party is at significant risk (e.g. the partner of an HIV-positive patient, who is unaware of the diagnosis and risk).

Consent and confidentiality go hand in hand, and it is good practice to seek the patient's consent to disclosure of any information wherever possible, whether or not you judge that a patient can be identified from the disclosure.

The Human Rights Act (1998), the Data Protection Act (1998), the Crime Disorder Act (1998) and the Common Law Duty of confidence all enable agencies to share information without consent with regard to children at risk of harm. Any person arguing that their medical information has been unlawfully disclosed is likely to argue the right to private life (Article 8(1) of the Human Rights Act).

Access to Health Records Act (1990)

A patient has the right to see their medical records, obtain copies of these records and have records explained.

Limitations include the following.

● This act only applies to records after 1 November 1991. Records before this date are included if they are needed to understand later notes.

- A doctor can deny access to a patient's medical records if they believe serious harm to the patient's physical or mental health will result from seeing those records.
- A doctor should ensure that confidentiality of other individuals is maintained.

The doctor's duties in accessing health records

- The doctor should enable the patient to see the records (or copies) within 21 days, or 40 days for records that are more than 40 days old.
- The doctor may charge a reasonable fee for copying records and time spent explaining records.
- The doctor should make appropriate corrections if the original data are incorrect.

Confidentiality and the Caldicott Report

The Caldicott Report was issued following the review of patient-identifiable information by the Caldicott Committee in December 1997.

The report was commissioned in light of the publication of *The Protection and Use of Patient Information* in 1996, due to concerns about the way patient information is used in the NHS and the need to ensure confidentiality is not undermined.

There are 16 recommendations (www.doh.gov.uk/confiden/crep.htm):

1 Every data flow, current or proposed, should be tested against basic principles of good practice. Continuing flows should be retested regularly.

2 A programme of work should be established to reinforce awareness of confidentiality and information security requirements among all staff within the NHS.

3 A senior person, preferably a health professional, should be nominated in each health organisation to act as a guardian who is responsible for safeguarding the confidentiality of patient information.

4 Clear guidance should be provided for those individuals/bodies responsible for approving uses of patient-identifiable information.

5 Protocols should be developed to protect the exchange of patient-identifiable information between NHS and non-NHS bodies.

6 The identity of those responsible for monitoring the sharing and transfer of information within agreed local protocols should be clearly communicated.

7 An accreditation system which recognises those organisations following good practice with respect to confidentiality should be considered.

8 The NHS number should replace all other identifiers wherever practicable, taking account of the consequences of errors and particular requirements for other specific identifiers.

9 Strict protocols should define who is authorised to gain access to patient identity where the NHS number or other coded identifier is used.

10 In cases where particularly sensitive information is transferred, privacy-enhanced technologies (e.g. encrypting identifiers or 'patient-identifying information') must be explored.

11 Those involved in developing health information systems should ensure that best practice principles are incorporated during the design stage.

12 Where practicable, the internal structure and administration of databases holding patient-identifiable information should reflect the principles developed in this report.

13 The NHS number should replace the patient's name on Items-of-Service claims made by GPs as soon as is practically possible.

14 The design of new systems for transfer of prescription data should incorporate the principles developed in the Caldicott Report.

15 Future negotiations on pay and conditions for GPs should, where possible, avoid systems of payment which require patient-identifying details to be transmitted.

16 Consideration should be given to procedures for GP claims and payments which do not require patient-identifying information to be transferred, which can then be piloted.

If you only remember five points from the Caldicott guidelines try to remember that information should be:

- held securely and confidentially
- obtained fairly and efficiently
- recorded accurately and reliably
- used effectively and efficiently
- shared appropriately and lawfully.

Freedom of Information Act 2000

www.foi.nhs.uk

This Act came into force on 1 January 2005. It means that GPs (as well as other public services) are obliged to respond to requests for information that is held (in any format) within 20 days (although this is negotiable at the time of request). A fee is not usually charged for any work that needs to be carried out to produce the information but where a fee is appropriate, there is a limit of £450 per request.

There are penalties for non-compliance and failure to produce the information. The maximum penalty for a lead GP is two years imprisonment. Most practices will have prepared a publication scheme prior to the Act coming into force, so that a number of enquiries could be referred to the website.

There are 23 exemptions (reasons why information would not need to be supplied), which fulfil either of the following criteria.

- Absolute exemptions, e.g. court records, legal prohibition, information accessible by the applicant by other means, security issues, personal information and information provided in confidence.

- Public interest test, e.g. commercial interests (this includes your private income), environmental information, health and safety, audit results, internal relations and information intended for future publication.

General practitioner's workload

The Royal College of General Practitioners published its updated information sheet on GP workload in May 2001. Its findings can be summarised as follows.

- There has been an increase in the number of part-time contracts in general practice from 5.4% in 1990 to 18.4% in 2001.

- The number of hours worked for a full-time GP, when not on call, has increased marginally from 38.84 to 39.21 hours per week.

- The list size of the unrestricted principal has fallen over the last 13 years to around 1,665 patients.

- The number of consultations has fallen since 1983 from 8,335 to 8,030 per year.

- The number of home visits has decreased.

- The number of telephone consultations has increased marginally.

- Consultation length has increased from 8.4 to 9.36 minutes over the last 10 years.

How should hamsters run? Some observations about sufficient patient time in primary care
BMJ 2001; 323: 206–8

This article summarises that GPs in the UK and the USA believe they have less time for each patient, although statistically this is not the case. Doctors in fact feel stressed because there is now more that can be done within a consultation and for a particular problem, patients' expectations are higher and there are more external forces impinging on their practice.

There is little evidence to support that doctors are 'running faster' in terms of both patient management and administration, despite the fact that doctors complain more. Reasons why areas of workload have increased are listed below.

- The population has increased by 3%, and is now 58.4 million (the birth rate is lower, so a large proportion of this increase is due to immigration).

- Life expectancy has doubled over the past 150 years:
  - there has been a 9% increase in the geriatric population in the past decade
  - there has been a 13% increase in the population aged over 75 years in the past decade.

- The number of infant deaths has decreased.

- Divorce affects one in two marriages (with associated social morbidity).

- Families are more spread out (i.e. there is a decreased support network).

- There are more single-parent families.

- Preventative healthcare has added 23% to the workload.

- It is now more acceptable to present with mental health problems.

- Most consultations are minor; 15% are life-threatening and need to be identified.

- Overall knowledge has increased (the *Oxford Textbook of Medicine* now runs to three volumes).

- There is increased accessibility (by telephone and email) to healthcare and surgeries.

- GPs are accountable for practice nurse roles, etc.

- Advances in information technology.

- There are more part-time GPs.

Wanless (a former NatWest Bank chief executive) has published his final report *Securing Our Future: taking a long-term view* (the Wanless Report). The main points can be summarised as follows.

- The current method of funding healthcare, through general taxation, is fair and efficient so should not be tampered with.

- Around 70% of work currently done by doctors could be done by nurses and other healthcare professionals.

- Medical services are being forced towards greater specialisation.

The new GMS contract (2004) was partly sold as a way in which GPs could control their workload. However, there are significant penalties for doctors choosing to limit certain services. There are many initiatives to try and ease workload, such as electronic prescribing, nurse practitioners and prescribers, and nursing management for chronic disease reviews. Similarly, there are many issues that will demand an increase in our workload in the future, such as Choose and Book, and practice-based commissioning. What is always important in managing workload is a person's personal work ethic and their time management skills.

Stress and burnout

There are four levels of human functioning: emotional, mental, behavioural and psychological.

Burnout is the end-stage response to excessive stress and dissatisfaction. No one is immune to stress, and you need to find a work pressure level that is constructive, not destructive. To do this, you need to be self-aware and able to recognise how it affects you. How you then manage will depend on whether you think the level of stress is a good or a bad thing. It should be actively managed with your own personal survival plan to prevent burnout in the long term.

Stress is also a physiological response to an inappropriate level of pressure. Noradrenaline levels increase and this, via the medulla, increases adrenaline production. This in turn increases ACTH levels and hence steroid production, which we all know improves immunity and ability to deal with stress. When you stop working or go on holiday, all this falls apart and you develop a cold!

People heading towards burnout go through four stages: overwork, frustration, resentment and finally depression (with burnout). It has always been acceptable to complain about stress, but it has not been acceptable to have symptoms, as these are interpreted as a sign of weakness. As GPs we need to be aware of the wellbeing of our employees and ourselves.

Causes of stress

These include the following:

- escalating workload
- frequently imposed change
- patients' expectations
- fear of litigation
- conflict (e.g. between career and family life)
- lack of career structure, etc.

Predisposing features

In the doctor, these include the following:

- type A personality, obsessional personality
- conscientiousness, high personal standards
- reluctance to decline work
- reluctance to delegate
- competitive nature
- fear of failure to match colleagues' achievements.

In the practice, they include the following:

- single-handed or dysfunctional partnership
- professional isolation
- repeated interruptions

- unpredictable work
- long hours, out-of-hours cover
- lack of variety, no challenge
- lack of peer recognition.

In society, predisposing features include the following:

- increased patient expectation
- shift of work from secondary care
- increasing litigation and complaints
- imposed change and political agendas.

Signs of stress and burnout to look out for include the following:

- poor time keeping and decision making
- sick leave
- increasing frequency of mistakes
- strained relationships.

What can we do for our employees?

- Understand that inappropriate pressures lead to stress; differentiate between pressure and stress.
- Conduct staff appraisals/personal development plans to identify problems.
- Hold practice development sessions:
  - review attitudes to stress
  - audit – establish a baseline, make the issue less confrontational, measure effectiveness of any strategy
  - develop skills at dealing with pressure – assertiveness (not aggression) and increase resilience – by creating a balance and developing your own strategy for dealing with pressure
  - look at neurolinguistic programming – this technique helps you to understand the structure of how you think and behave; it uses specific techniques to make your thinking and behaviour more resourceful.
- Be vigilant, observe individuals.
- Develop your own helping skills.
- Useful websites:
  - www.mindtools.com
  - www.employersforwork-lifebalance.org.uk.

What can we do to avoid burnout ourselves?
Br J Gen Pract **1993; 43(376): 442–3**

This article made the following recommendations.

- Trainees should be given realistic expectations of general practice.
- Choose the right job.
- Develop practice support systems as well as personal ones (e.g. groups outside work).
- Be assertive.
- Develop time-management skills.
- Be aware of your own response to stress.

Other considerations

Delegate, prioritise, keep up to date, audit, develop practice policies, balance your life (maintain outside interests) and make sure you have a plan for dealing with stress. Organise your workload with realistic targets. Also take time out to exercise and for other hobbies (i.e. strike a professional/personal balance).

MedNet is a service that allows doctors who may feel that the profession is not right for them to explore other options. The service can offer some sessions to reflect on how the medical role and work impact on the personal struggles of a doctor. They can be contacted on Tel: 020 7447 3790 or at www.londondeanery.co.uk.

How you manage pressure, stress or burnout is up to you, but make sure you do manage it, otherwise someone will take it in hand and you will be 'managed' as someone else deems appropriate – not a comfortable situation.

The difficult patient

This is an inevitable problem for us all, and it happens for different reasons (doctor, patient and/or external factors). Heartsink patients represent a different group of people to frequent attenders. They have been defined (by Groves, 1978) as patients who most physicians would dread having to treat as they engender negative feelings.

As early as 1951, Groves defined four types of difficult patient:

1 *Dependent clinger* – grateful, but seeking reassurance for minor ailments.

2 *Entitled demander* – complaining about imagined shortcomings in the service provided.

3 *Manipulative health rejector* – has symptoms that the doctor cannot improve.

4 *Self-destructive denier* – refuses to accept that their behaviour affects their illness and will not modify their habits.

Heartsink patients are often over-investigated or referred unnecessarily, particularly if they are seeing several GPs and no one doctor takes responsibility for that patient.

It is important, for your own sanity (as well as being in the patient's best interest), to develop coping strategies and a sensible, thorough approach to heartsink patients.

Coping strategies

- Recognise your own feelings.
- Accept that heartsinks will occur.
- Review the patient's notes.
- Set goal limits for the patient.
- Assume ownership of a problem and review it regularly.
- Set limits for the patient (e.g. when you expect to see them again).
- Challenge inappropriate demands.
- Hold peer group meetings/Balint groups with other doctors.
- Consider alternative sources of therapy for the patient.

Heartsink patients: a study of their general practitioners
Br J Gen Pract 1995; 45(395): 293–6

Mathers looked at the heartsink patients' GPs and found that GPs who had a low level of job satisfaction and no postgraduate qualifications reported more heartsink patients. It is important to recognise this association – for our own self-preservation. If we are stressed, our coping mechanisms start to fail and we start heading towards burnout.

Chronic disease management

Chronic diseases are the main cause of morbidity and mortality in developed countries (having overtaken infectious diseases), and they account for almost a quarter of GPs' workload, according to recent statistics. Managing these conditions effectively helps to reduce complications and deterioration, avert a potential crisis, and reduce acute admission and referral rates to secondary care.

Meeting the needs of chronically ill people
BMJ 2001; 323: 945–6 (Editorial)

This editorial reiterated that the best outcomes depend on competent self-management and decision making by patients, as well as clinical treatments. It also brings to the forefront the frequent co-occurrence of mental disorders.

The elements of a chronic disease management programme usually include the following:

- clinical guidelines
- patient-friendly information which is accessible
- continuous quality improvement and clinical audit
- access to specialist care
- resource management techniques and systems
- case management
- patient education and counselling
- tracking systems
- national disease registers.

Having chronic disease morbidity registers allows audit of standards such as compliance and prescribing. This in turn enables better planning of services and necessary changes. The data extracted are dependent on accuracy of diagnosis and coding. A number of chronic diseases form part of the specific indicators in the new GMS contract.

Further issues

- Care must be organised. If a system is methodical it reduces the risk of error. The use of computers is very helpful both in terms of speed (once the data have been input) and for audit when trying to improve quality. Protocols need to be in place, but flexible enough to allow for patient-dependent factors.

- The patient should be the most important member of the team. It is their life and in essence we are there in an advisory capacity.

- Ethical issues arise when giving the patient a diagnosis of a chronic disease and then motivating them with regard to management and compliance, when they still consider themselves to be a 'normal healthy adult'.

- Economic and political issues arise in funding screening programmes and chronic disease clinics in an evidence-based way (medical care, equipment, administration, audit, etc.).

- No doctor or other member of the primary healthcare team should make the mistake of underestimating the psychological impact that a chronic disease can have on a person's life. It should not be trivialised, but wherever possible we should endeavour to help that person to keep things in perspective.

The Expert Patient: a new approach to chronic disease management in the 21st century, published in 2001, proposed that every primary care group should have a lay-led training course in self-management of chronic diseases for patients. A total of £2 million is being invested in the pilot schemes and to mainstream the programmes through the NHS by 2007.

Although individual patients have needs specific to their particular disease, they have a core of common requirements:

- knowing how to recognise and act upon symptoms
- dealing with acute attacks or exacerbations of the disease
- making the most effective use of medicines and treatment
- understanding the implications of professional advice
- establishing a stable pattern of sleep and rest, and dealing with fatigue
- accessing social and other services
- managing work and resources of employment services
- accessing chosen leisure activities
- developing strategies to deal with the psychological consequence of illness
- learning to cope with other people's response to their chronic illness.

Monitoring chronic disease: a rational approach
BMJ 2005; 330: 644–8 (Clinical Review)

This is an interesting review taking the reader through the phases of monitoring in chronic disease and the importance of measuring the correct marker (for predicting clinical outcome and detecting changes in risk early). It considers monitoring a patient for both benefit and harm (in response to treatment), and the fact that although we always try to monitor progress, it may not always be beneficial to the patient.

Labelling chronic disease in primary care: a good or a bad thing?
Br J Gen Pract 2004; 54: 932–8

This discussion paper specifically considers osteoarthritis. It considers that diagnostic labels are useful when symptoms relate to pathology (which in turn can help with decisions on effective management), but emphasises that labels have limitations and can overstate a problem, which may misdirect a patient's perception.

Guidelines

Guidelines are defined as systematically developed statements to assist practitioner and patient in making decisions about appropriate healthcare for specific clinical circumstances (Field and Lohr).

The aims of producing guidelines are as follows:

- to assist decision making
- to improve quality of care, effectiveness and outcome
- to standardise medical practice.

Guidelines need to be produced in an evidence-based way that acknowledges limitations such as resources, staffing and the local population for whom the guidelines are intended. They are thought of as a simple way of getting evidence out into practice.

Guidelines in practice, considering their role

Are they useful?

- Are they relevant in a clinical context?
- Are they user friendly?
- Are they evidence based?

Appraisal of guidelines takes place through the NHS Appraisal Centre for Clinical Guidelines prior to national implementation.

Implementation

- The people who will be using the guidelines should have a sense of ownership, and should preferably be involved in the development (if not, then they should be involved in auditing and making amendments at a later stage).
- Local facilitators should help with the process of implementation.

Legal implications

- Guidelines can be used in court by an expert witness (but not in place of the latter) to demonstrate standards of care.
- Non-compliance with clinical guidelines does not mean that care is sub-standard.

Compliance

It can be difficult to comply with guidelines as they are not written for individual patients, but rather they reflect a consensus opinion based on the current evidence without making it apparent that they take into account uncertainties and ethical or cultural issues that may arise in clinical management.

Potential benefits of guidelines

Benefits for patients include the following:

- improved consistency of care
- empowerment to make informed choices.

Benefits for healthcare professionals include the following:

- improved quality of clinical decisions (although to a variable degree)
- they are evidence based so improve knowledge, highlight gaps and through audit improve quality of care.

Benefits for healthcare systems include the following:

- efficient use of resources
- distributive justice (i.e. ethical issues relating to rationing)
- improved public perception of equality.

Potential drawbacks of guidelines

- They may be incorrect/flawed/biased or conflict with other professional groups.
- They can be time-consuming to implement.
- They are written for populations, not individuals.
- They will increase the overall resources needed (e.g. statins in cardiovascular disease).
- They need regular review to keep them up to date and usable.
- They do not address the complexity and uncertainties of medical practice.
- There are a vast number in use that we must be familiar with.

Quality of care of older patients with multiple co-morbid conditions: implications for pay performance
JAMA 2005; 294: 716–24

This paper looked at following guidelines for major conditions (hypertension, ischaemic heart disease, diabetes, COPD and osteoarthritis) in a hypothetical case and found that although the hypothetical patient would be eligible for 12 medications, none of the guidelines modified their directives or discussed issues relating to co-morbidity.

Developing clinical guidelines: a challenge to current methods
BMJ 2005; 331: 631–3 (Education and Debate)

This is an interesting view discussing the drawbacks of the current publication of guidelines (lack of consensus, transparency and failure to make clear the level of resources we have in the health system). It explains the three most commonly used methods of developing guidelines (nominal group technique, the Delphi survey and a hybrid of the two) and suggests a way forward, which would enhance transparency by having explicit guideline goals, providing information on reasons for disagreement and including information on the strength of support for the recommendation.

Screening

Wilson's criteria (1966) can be briefly summarised as follows.

1 The condition must be:
   - common
   - important
   - diagnosable by acceptable methods.

2 There should be a latent period where effective interventional treatment is possible.

3 Screening must be:
   - cheap/cost-effective
   - continuous
   - safe
   - repeatable
   - non-invasive
   - acceptable to patients
   - such that the test for screening has a high positive predictive value.

4 Treatment must be available.

Technically, screening is a form of secondary prevention, i.e. it involves identifying pre-symptomatic disease before significant damage is done. Examples of primary prevention would include immunisation and water sanitation. Tertiary prevention is about limiting complications (e.g. in diabetic care).

When establishing a screening programme you need to consider not just the ethics of the test, but also the implications of positive and false-positive results. An increasing number of studies are looking at the negative effects of screening. For example a normal cholesterol result may mean that a patient's diet subsequently lapses because they feel justified in indulging more often. Another example would be the psychological implications of being given a positive result after, say, chlamydia screening.

The UK National Screening Committee is responsible for advising the Government on the merits of screening for a particular disease and health problems. It published its first report in 1998 and the second in 2000. In the final section of the report it set out recommendations for eight common conditions: aortic aneurysms, diabetic retinopathy, vascular disease, osteoporosis, hypertrophic cardiomyopathy, ovarian cancer, prostate cancer and syphilis.

Gaining informed consent. Is difficult – but many misconceptions need to be undone
BMJ 1999; 319: 722–3 (Editorial)

The author discussed some of the detrimental effects of screening, such as anxiety, false alarms, false reassurance, unnecessary biopsies and associated risk, over-diagnosis and over-treatment. Because of these implications, the issues relating to obtaining consent, emphasising the importance of sharing decision making and a patient's autonomy, are of paramount importance and should be considered.

Medicine and the Internet

It is accepted that the Internet can improve communication and access both among professionals and with patients.

Cybermedicine
BMJ 1999; 319: 1294–6

An estimated 25 million people use the Internet to access health information, of whom 27% are female and 15% are male. [*sic*]

One of the biggest problems with information on the net is that there is no quality control/regulation (i.e. there is no guarantee that the information is reliable), which means that as GPs we may need to guide our patients. Health on the Net (www.hon.ch/) is an international organisation which provides a database of evaluated health material. Any website health information which displays the HON logo was developed in accordance with the foundation's guidelines. Worldwide online Reliable Advice to Patients and Individuals (WRAPIN) has been developed to enable comparison of health/medical documents in any format with this interconnected knowledge base, another step towards the certification of quality online information.

NHSnet

As part of the Government directive, all GP practices should be connected to NHSnet. It is planned that health records will be networked, thus allowing doctors 24-hour access. Inevitably, this raises data protection issues, which are addressed in the Caldicott Report 1999. Appointment (Choose and Book), X-ray and pathology requests will be made online, and pharmacists will accept prescriptions electronically.

The potential applications of NHSnet are limited only by us. At whatever speed things are implemented, the systems used need to have been thought through in terms of confidentiality (patient and doctor), data protection and litigation issues. They also need to be quick, user-friendly and accurate.

The National Programme for IT (www.doh.gov.uk) is being implemented across the UK. The goal is to improve access to information and to develop more traceable service activity within the NHS.

There are several major changes that should improve our ability to deliver for our patients. The main ones are listed below.

- Clinical records – will be available to out-of-hours doctors and will be jointly used by those professionals caring for patients (this should allow us to make better clinical decisions and reduce risk). By 2008, it is anticipated that Health Space will allow patients to read their own records.

- Electronic prescribing – repeat prescribing will be managed by pharmacists rather than being requested through GPs. Again this should improve satisfaction and safety. It should also reduce the number of fraudulent scripts.

- Administration – booking online (Choose and Book) for hospital and GP appointments.

European Computer Driving Licence (ECDL) Programme

This is a scheme to allow all NHS staff to train online and be examined to ECDL standards, over seven modules of basic skills.

The scheme was developed in Finland in 1988, and over 200,000 people in the UK are now registered.

More information is available at www.nhsia.nhs.uk.

Evidence-based medicine

Evidence-based medicine (EBM) was coined as a buzz phrase in the early 1990s, and has increased our awareness of research studies and improved our knowledge base within the profession as a whole. This can give our patients the confidence that we are up to date and giving them appropriate advice.

Research findings (the evidence) are almost never black and white, and often only look at a specific point at the expense of other issues (e.g. resources) in a specific clinical environment. This leaves us the clinicians (who are not the best at interpreting studies) with the dilemma of how – or indeed if – we should use certain findings.

Why GPs do not implement evidence: qualitative study
BMJ 2001; 323: 1100–2

This article considered why GPs are generally cautious about the evidence-based model. They are reluctant to jeopardise relationships with patients, and patients are often unwilling to take certain drugs. It concluded that GPs regarded clinical evidence as a square peg to be fitted into the round hole of a patient's life. The process of implementation is complex, fluid and adaptive.

Providing education on evidence-based practice improved knowledge but did not change behaviour
BMC Med Educ 2005; 5(1): 40

This study of 114 self-selected occupational therapists starts by acknowledging that our skills as health professionals do not naturally encompass appraisal of published research. They found that although changes in behaviour were seen with targeted intervention and outreach support (adapted Fresno Test of 1.2 points, 95% CI −6.0 to 8.5), they were small. It is recognised that behaviour changes take months and must include new routines and priorities which could be developed in the workplace, probably more effectively than in a workshop setting.

Sources of evidence are diverse, but the gold standard is held to be a meta-analysis of randomised controlled trials. The Cochrane Reviews are one point at which to access some such information, although their validity has been questioned.

Quality of Cochrane Reviews: assessment of sample from 1998
BMJ 2001; 323: 829–32

This review concluded that although the Cochrane database is a key source of evidence, users should interpret reviews cautiously, especially where experimental interventions are advocated. In nine out of 53 reviews it was found that the evidence did not support the conclusions.

The Cochrane Collaboration has taken steps to improve the quality of its reviews following the minor problems highlighted by this study.

DARE (Database of Abstracts of Reviews of Effects) is another tool forming part of the Cochrane Library which contains systematic reviews. This can be accessed free of charge at www.york.ac.uk/inst/crd/crddatabase.htm, or alternatively you can telephone 01904 433707 and someone will conduct the search for you.

Validation of the Fresno test of competence in EBM
BMJ 2003; 236: 319–21

This test was developed by the Fresno Medical Education Programme in California. It is a tool for assessing knowledge and skill (ability) in teaching evidence-based medicine and can identify the strengths and weaknesses of curricula and individuals. It has a standardised grading system and seems to be valid, although the authors point out that familiarity may have led to unrealistic scoring.

Death certification

Death certification provides legal evidence of the fact and cause(s) of death, which then allows the death to be registered. It has been a statutory obligation in England since the 1830s. It is important to be as accurate as possible – a mode of dying is not acceptable as the cause of death.

Terms that imply a mode of dying include the following:

- asphyxia
- asthenia
- brain failure
- cachexia
- cardiac arrest
- cardiac failure
- coma
- debility

- exhaustion
- hepatic failure
- renal failure
- respiratory arrest
- shock
- syncope
- uraemia
- vagal inhibition.

Old age can only be used as a cause of death if the person is over 70 years of age and a more specific cause of death cannot be given.
   Duties of the medical practitioner of the deceased include the following.

- If you were in attendance in the deceased's last illness, you are required to certify the cause of death.
- You are legally responsible for the delivery of the death certificate to the registrar. This may be done in person, by post or by a relative (or other person).
- You should also complete the notice to informant (attached to the death certificate) and the counterfoil in the book for your records.

There are three types of certificate.

- Medical Certificate of cause of death (Form 66) – for any death after the first 28 days of life.
- Neonatal Death Certificate (Form 65) – for any live-born death within 28 days of birth.
- Certificate of Stillbirth (Form 34) – for any death of an infant after 34 weeks of pregnancy which showed no signs of life after delivery from the mother.

When to refer to the coroner

There is no statutory duty to report to the coroner (this would otherwise be done by the registrar), but voluntary reporting where suggested avoids unnecessary delay and anxiety for the relatives.
   A death should be referred if:

- the cause of death is unknown
- the deceased has not been seen by the certifying doctor either after death or within 14 days before death

- death was violent, unnatural or suspicious

- the death may be due to an accident (whenever it occurred)

- the death may be due to self-neglect or neglect by others

- the death may be due to industrial disease or related to the deceased's employment

- the death may be due to an abortion

- the death occurred during an operation or before recovery from the effects of an anaesthetic

- the death may be suicide

- the death occurred during, or shortly after, detention in police or prison custody.

Death certification and doctors' dilemmas: a qualitative study of GPs' perspectives
Br J Gen Pract 2005; 55: 677–83

This paper gives a good introduction to the additional uses of death certification:

- to monitor trends and patterns of disease

- to guide health promotion, resource allocation and service planning

- for research and epidemiology

- for the settlement of estates, welfare and pensions entitlements.

Inaccuracies of death certification are thought to range from 20 to 65%, and when looking at determining influences on the recording of a cause of death it was found that clinical uncertainty and the role of the deceased's family were the two main themes.

The Shipman Inquiry

www.doh.gov.uk

The Shipman Inquiry was set up in January 2001 following the conviction of Harold Shipman for the murder of 15 of his patients. Its purpose was to investigate the extent of Shipman's unlawful activities, enquire into the activities of statutory authorities and other organisations involved, and to then make recommendations on steps needed to protect patients in the future.

Five reports have been published by Dame Janet Smith and her team. The first three look at the extent of Shipman's criminal activities (looking into the care of more than 800 patients), the police investigation and death certification. The fourth report (*The Regulation of Controlled Drugs in the Community*, published in July 2004) gives a detailed report on prescribing, dispensing, storing and disposing of controlled drugs. The fifth report (*Safeguarding Patients: lessons from the past – proposals for the future*, published in December 2004) looks at revalidation and monitoring of GP performance, the role of the GMC, disciplinary procedures, whistle blowing and the handling of complaints.

Recommendations for death certification include the following.

- A coroner's office should be notified of all deaths.

- The officer should examine two forms before certifying the cause of death:
  - Form 1 – completed by a health professional recording the facts surrounding death, including the persons present at the time of death
  - Form 2 – to be completed by the doctor who last treated the patient; relevant sections of the patient's notes could be attached.

A practical method for monitoring general practice mortality in the UK: findings from a pilot study in a health board of Northern Ireland
Br J Gen Pract 2005; 55: 670–6

Monitoring mortality rates was recommended in the Baker Report, following the Shipman case. This would pose several challenges. The data would need to be of a high quality, and be linked to general practices. It is not clear how easy it would be to distinguish variations in mortality and, if any variation was identified, what should be done with the information. This pilot study looked at cross-sectional and longitudinal mortality rate variations and assigning variation reasons (e.g. nursing homes, levels of deprivation, age/sex profiles). The ultimate aim of the data collection in the pilot was to improve quality of care. There was a consensus of apprehension about the release of any such data to the public and how it might be incorrectly interpreted.

Recommendations for revalidation include the following.

- A mandatory knowledge-based test at least every 7 years, every 5 years if the clinician is over 50 years of age.

- It should include a folder of mandatory evidence (e.g. prescribing data, complaints record, evidence of continuing professional development).

- Primary care trusts would be able to issue warnings and impose financial penalties to underperforming GPs.

Concerns raised about the GMC include the following.

- There has been a failure to lay down clear policies governing fitness to practise procedures.

- There has been a failure to take into account the difficulties faced by complainants.

- There has been a failure to investigate complaints.

- There has been a tendency to preserve a doctor's privacy against the legitimate public interest.

- There is a concern over determination to undertake a sufficiently thorough investigation.

GMC and the future of revalidation
BMJ 2005; 330: 1205–7

This article is written by Graham Catto, in a positive light, looking at the lessons that can be taken from the inquiry, and where parts of the system can be strengthened and improved upon. He also makes criticisms about where the mark was overstepped, in that little regard was given to the context of the GMC's many other roles.

Advance directives (living wills)

In medieval times a good death was a prepared death. Advance directives are statements (usually written and formally witnessed) made by a person about the medical care that they do and do not want if they become incompetent in the future.

Is there such a thing as a life not worth living?
BMJ 2001; 322: 1481–3

This article debates the practical difficulties of measurement, and ethical issues associated with, determining quality of life in situations where a life has been judged to have no quality. Patients who are dying may find some quality in life even when it has been assessed by current measures as abysmal. The use of proxies is touched on as a problem for similar reasons, namely the disparity between an observer's assessment and the patient's own evaluation.

Legally, the whole subject of advance directives is complicated. At present there are six types of advance statements:

1 a requesting statement reflecting an individual's aspirations and preferences

2 a statement of general beliefs and aspects of life that the individual values

3 a statement naming proxy

4 a directive giving clear instructions relating to some or all of treatment

5 a statement specifying a degree of irreversible deterioration after which no life-sustaining treatment should be given

6 a combination of all of the above.

An advance directive should not preclude the provision of basic care, defined as maintenance of bodily cleanliness, relief of sustained pain, and provision of oral nutrition and hydration.

The current legal situation in the UK

- The person must be competent at the time of declaration (Mental Capacity Act 2005).

- The person must be informed in broad terms about the nature and effect of treatments and procedures.

- The person must have anticipated and intended the refusal to apply to the circumstances that subsequently arise.

- The person must be free from undue influence when issuing the declaration.

Advance directives in the UK: legal, ethical and practical considerations
BMJ 1998; 48: 1263–6

This paper highlights the fact that most articles written on the subject cover legal or practical matters, and it points out that it is not in the best interest of the doctor or patient to reduce medical ethics to medical law.

Adherence to advance directives in critical care decision making: vignette study
BMJ 2003; 327: 1011–14

This article raises the point that advance directives are open to widely varying interpretation, partly due to the ambiguity of a directive's terminology, and partly due to the willingness of health professionals to make value judgements concerning quality of life.

A GP is likely to be involved with advance directives in one of two ways:

1 advising patients when advance directives may be appropriate and advising on the phrasing of the directive (visitors to the Age Concern website, www.ageconcern. org.uk, can obain information on advance directives and a pack to help draw up a directive)

2 as a repository of the advance directive, which could be forwarded to the appropriate department on request.

An advance directive has been legally binding on a doctor in common law since 1994, and has been endorsed by the British Medical Association since 1995 and the legal professions. Most experts believe that directives should be reviewed periodically (e.g. every 5 years).

Formatted versions are available from either the Terrence Higgins Trust (020 7831 0330) or the Voluntary Euthanasia Society (020 7937 7770).

Medic Alert is allowed to engrave bracelets advising that the patient has a living will, and can also keep a copy and fax it to the appropriate department or read it to the paramedics.

Withholding and withdrawing life-prolonging treatments. Good practice in decision making
General Medical Council August 2002, www.gmc-uk.org
This publication looks at guiding principles and our ethical obligations to show respect for human life, dilemmas of starting and stopping treatment, a framework of good practice, and areas of special consideration. Your revision of this area would not be complete without reading this.

Assisted dying and euthanasia

Both assisted dying and euthanasia involve medical assistance. Providing a patient with the means to end life (e.g. medication) is termed *physician-assisted suicide*, while ending the life of a patient who is physically unable to do so themselves is termed *voluntary euthanasia*. Both are illegal in the UK, and a World Medical Association resolution has condemned the practices as unethical. At the BMA's annual meeting in 2005, a vote was carried to allow parliament and society to decide on the issue of assisted dying.

Moral dimensions
BMJ 2005; 331:689–91 (Education and Debate)

The author considers the following three moral outlooks:

- *deontology* – the view that some kinds of action are unconditionally prohibited, the sanctity of life doctrine is often the argument against euthanasia
- *basic (negative) moral rights* – meaning that individuals are free to do as they see fit with themselves. With this view we have no positive right to receive help when we are in distress
- *utilitarianism* – an action is wrong if, and only if, an alternative is available with better consequences.

Although many doctors and politicians oppose legalised euthanasia, this article concludes that in limited circumstances it may be beneficial.

Taking the final step: changing the law on euthanasia and physician-assisted suicide
BMJ 2005; 331:681–3 (Education and Debate)

This is written from a legal perspective and opens with a profound statement: doctors in the UK can accompany their patients every step of the way, up until the last. The law stops them helping their patients take the final step. The proposed legislation under the Assisted Dying for the Terminally Ill Bill, would allow a competent adult (who has lived in the UK for at least one year), who is suffering unbearably as a result of a terminal illness, to receive medical assistance to die at his or her request. The bill includes various safeguards to protect both the patient and the physician. Current public opinion is 82% in favour of allowing assisted dying.

Many concerns are discussed following the above paper. They look at the Oregon model of assisted suicide (1997 law allowing doctors to end the life of their terminally ill patients where requested by the patient), legalisation in Sweden and the need for patients to travel when they are at one of the most vulnerable points in life (for themselves and their family), often in pain. Similarly the worries doctors have if they were to consider undertaking such a role and the impact on their own personal and religious beliefs. Although the bill may go some way to addressing these concerns and providing a legal framework, the issues will continue to be debated at length.

Assisted suicide and euthanasia in Switzerland: allowing a role for non-physicians
BMJ 2003; 326: 271–3

This is an educational publication. Assisted suicide is not a criminal act under Swiss law, but a physician's professional ethics could lead to a personal conflict about assisting death. Altruistic assisted suicide by non-physicians is legal in Switzerland, which has enabled certain issues to be separated, but the whole debate will continue.

The House of Lords Select Committee has recently been asked to consider the Assisted Dying for the Terminally Ill Bill, and the US courts have recently concluded that doctors can lawfully withdraw hydration and nutrition from a patient in a vegetative state. This, and the fact that we have improved our life span (through public health and improved medical care), and increased knowledge of human rights and the limitations of modern technologies, mean that interest in assisted dying, in the media and society, has increased.

Integrated/alternative medicine

Complementary medicine (which focuses on health and healing) and conventional medicine (which focuses on disease and treatment) have traditionally been distinct from one another, but recently they have become increasingly integrated. This means that complementary medicine will have to be subject to similar clinical, scientific and regulatory standards to those applied to conventional healthcare.

The ABC of Complementary Medicine estimates that 30% of the UK population use alternative medicines and 40% of GPs offer access to complementary treatment.

Public awareness and use of complementary medicine have increased dramatically over the last 10 years, but many complementary practitioners remain unregulated. Osteopaths and chiropractors are now becoming the exception in the UK.

Regulating herbal medicines in the UK
BMJ 2005; 331: 62–3 (Editorial)

This editorial discusses the use of a specific committee to help consumers distinguish between unproved herbal therapies as compared to more pharmaceutical treatments proven to have an effect. Currently in the UK, the Medicines and Healthcare Products Regulatory Agency is consulting on a proposal for a herbal medicines committee.

Perceptions about complementary therapies relative to conventional therapies among adults who use both: results from a national survey
Ann Intern Med 2001; 135: 344–51

A total of 831 people in the USA who use alternative/complementary medicine were surveyed.

• Around 80% thought the combination of both complementary and conventional medicine was superior to either alone.

- Most saw a conventional doctor first.

- Around 70% did not subsequently disclose that they were seeing a complementary therapist as it was not thought to be any of the doctor's business, rather than this information being withheld for fear of criticism.

Acupuncture

On the basis of current evidence, acupuncture is effective in treating nausea and vomiting, back pain, dental pain and migraine. The incidence of adverse reactions to acupuncture is relatively low. It is the most popular form of complementary therapy among GPs (used by 47%). This popularity has only emerged in the UK over the past 20 years, although the technique has been used for many thousands of years in Chinese medicine.

Non-medical acupuncturists should be members of the British Acupuncture Council, which has strict educational criteria and a code of practice. Physiotherapists may belong to the Acupuncture Association of Chartered Physiotherapists.

Adverse events following acupuncture: prospective survey of 32,000 consultations with doctors and physiotherapists
BMJ 2001; 323: 485–6 (there is an accompanying editorial)

This study found that no adverse events were reported after 34,407 acupuncture treatments from data collected over a 4-week period. It did not look at patients' experiences of adverse events, but it is nevertheless encouraging and reassuring research.

Herbal remedies

The Traditional Herbal Products Directive came into force in October 2005. It means that all unlicensed herbal remedies sold in the UK will be regulated by 2011. Companies will have to prove that new products have a traditional use and have accompanying safety data.

Again popularity in the UK means sales are increasing by 20% a year. The users often have the belief that 'herbal equals natural', and that it is both safe and cheaper than conventional medicine, with no side effects. However, many herbal products do have side effects and can interact with other drugs.

As there is little legislation for control, doses of preparations can vary widely, even in the same product. Some products may also contain conventional medicines (e.g. one eczema cream was recently found to contain high doses of dexamethasone, although it had been advertised as a natural product).

- *Ginseng* – this is teratogenic, increases the international normalised ratio (INR) and may also increase blood pressure. It also interacts with digoxin. There are several varieties. The active ingredients (ginsenosides) are antioxidants and enhance nitrate production.

- *St John's Wort* – (*see* section on depression, p. 40) this is a weak SSRI and antiviral drug. It is a liver-enzyme inducer, so may reduce the concentrations of digoxin, carbamazepine, warfarin and the oral contraceptive pill. It also interacts with several other drugs.

- *Ginkgo biloba* – (*see* section on dementia, p. 55) this is used to delay clinical progression of dementia. It is a potent inhibitor of platelet-activating factor so can increase the risk of bleeds (including intracerebral bleeding) in patients on aspirin or warfarin.

The herbal advice line is staffed by members of the National Institute of Medical Herbalists (www.nimh.org.uk). They can give advice on remedies, interactions, and use of herbal products in children and pregnancy. The line is open Monday to Friday 9am–1pm. Tel: 01392 426022.

Homeopathy

This needs to be distinguished from herbal remedies. Homeopathic remedies contain minute or non-existent amounts of the original substance and are prepared by successive dilutions.

Although to our knowledge there are insufficient randomised controlled trials to advocate the use of homeopathic treatments in specific conditions, many people report having benefited from them.

Are the clinical effects of homeopathy placebo effect? Comparative study of placebo controlled trials of homeopathy and allopathy
Lancet **2005; 366: 726–32**

This meta-analysis of 110 trials concluded that their results were not compatible with the hypothesis that the clinical effects of homeopathy were completely due to placebo effect. There was weak evidence for a specific effect of homeopathic remedies, but the findings were compatible with the notion that the effect was that of placebo.

Homeopathy – A Guide for GPs (from the Faculty of Homeopathy) describes a range of NHS services that are now available, and gives details on how GPs can refer patients.

The Glasgow and London Homeopathic Hospitals are the two leading bodies in research in this field, but funding is severely lacking. The Faculty of Homeopathy website (www.trusthomeopathy.org/faculty) is a good source of information.

Antioxidants

These include ginseng, β-carotene, vitamins C and E, minerals such as zinc and copper, flavonoids etc.

Most of the evidence available is in the form of cohort studies. As yet there seems to be insufficient evidence that taking antioxidants offers much in the way of benefit to healthy people.

Air travel

When booking our holidays and long-haul flights, few of us will give much thought to our health, but increasingly as GPs we will be asked questions about risk and recommendations for prevention of, for example, deep vein thrombosis (DVT).

In response to the House of Lords report on health and air travel (November 2000), the Department of Health has published advice for passengers (this can be found at www.doh.gov.uk/dvt).

The absolute risk of thrombosis is small. The longer the duration of travel, the higher the apparent risk, although there is no lower limit below which it is safe. As the risks for thrombosis are additive, short sequential flights probably increase the risk. Factors that put people at risk on long-haul flights include cramped conditions, varying air pressure and oxygen concentration, and dehydration (with or without excess alcohol consumption). Certain other factors put some people at higher risk than others, including obesity, heart disease, pregnancy, the pill, HRT, a family history of DVT, recent major leg surgery and increasing age.

Sensible advice is lacking in evidence, the general consensus is as follows:

- move around in the seat and in the cabin as much as possible

- rotate ankles and flex calf muscles regularly

- avoid alcohol and caffeine

- avoid dehydration (i.e. drink plenty of water).

Venous thromboembolic complications following air travel: what's the quantitative risk? A literature review
Eur J Vasc Endovasc Surg 2005; Oct 14

This was a limited study as there are few papers published on this subject. The authors found (from five papers) that there was a quantitative risk of 5% per flight for high-risk patients and 1.6% risk for low-risk patients, all following long-haul flights (longer than 8 hours).

TED stockings

Mediven travel stockings (which exert a pressure of 20 mmHg at the ankle) have been shown to reduce the incidence of DVT in travellers. There is no evidence for the effectiveness of lower-compression stockings.

Aspirin

The benefits of aspirin are arterial rather than venous. To my knowledge, no published study has shown any reduction in risk of thrombosis in travellers with aspirin use. It is important to be aware of the gastrointestinal risk, and that some clinics are advising taking 150 mg of aspirin the day before travel.

Subcutaneous heparin

This is indicated in high-risk patients, and it does reduce the risk of DVT. Usually, one injection 2–4 hours before travelling is adequate. If the patient is on warfarin there is no additional benefit.

Airogym

This is an inflatable cushion placed under the feet that simulates walking when pressed. The results so far are encouraging, but as yet there are no published outcome trials.

Medical ethics

> Understanding the law helps us deal with disputes, a proper understanding of medical ethics will help us work in true partnership with our patients.
> (Dr Cox, 8 November 2001)

This is a source of anxiety for many, especially when approaching exams like the MRCGP oral. The Hippocratic oath first outlined an ethical approach to medicine, and the General Medical Council requires that medical ethics be a core subject in the medical curriculum, and also that there should be a medical ethics curriculum. Try not to be daunted by the subject. Most of what you need you already know, but it is now a case of formulating a way of thinking and talking about ethical principles, using an ethical model that you can apply to a given situation.

Medical ethics applies to all areas of medicine, including end-of-life decisions, medical error, priority setting, biotechnology, education, consent and confidentiality.

Ethics and communication skills
Medicine **2000; 28**

This provides an excellent narrative, not just on ethics but on communication skills as well. I have summarised some of the discussion on ethics below.

Questions on ethical values cannot be solved by simply applying an algorithm. If we are to practise medicine in a way we think is right we must:

- clarify what value judgements are relevant in a specific clinical situation

- be aware of the relevant issues

- subject our views to critical analysis to ensure they are logical and consistent

- adapt or change our views in the light of such analysis.

In addition, we must practise medicine in a legal framework.

The Four Principles approach

This can be summarised as follows.

1 Respect for *autonomy* (self-rule) – help patients to make their own decisions and respect those decisions even when you do not agree with them.

2 *Beneficence* (do good) – this entails doing what is best for the patient, but who is the judge of what is best? This may conflict with autonomy.

3 *Non-maleficence* (avoiding harm) – in most cases this does not add anything to the principle of beneficence.

4 *Justice* – this incorporates time and resources.

Revising and implementing the Tavistock principles for everybody in health care
BMJ 2001; 323: 616–20

The Tavistock Group published their original five principles in 1999. The principles are not evidence based but are intended to serve as an ethical framework for those working to improve medical error.

The ethical concepts of the Tavistock Group

These can be summarised as follows.

- *Rights* – people have a right to health and healthcare.
- *Balance* – care of individual patients is central, but health of the population is also our concern.
- *Comprehensiveness* – in addition to treating illness we have an obligation to ease suffering, minimise disability, prevent disease and promote health.
- *Co-operation* – healthcare succeeds only if we co-operate with those we serve, each other and those in other sectors.
- *Improvement* – improving healthcare is a serious and continuing responsibility.
- *Safety* – do no harm.
- *Openness* – being open, honest and trustworthy is vital in healthcare.

The Declaration of Helsinki (revised for the fifth time by the World Medical Association) was adopted by the profession in 1964 and sets out widely accepted ethical principles for medical research involving human subjects. It is not clear whether this declaration has any real legal standing, or whether it is just to serve as a guide. The UK Clinical Ethics network is there to offer educational and practical support for clinical ethics groups. They are in place in around one-fifth of NHS trusts.

Consultation models

The consultation – you can't ignore it, it is central to what we do every single day. To be an effective doctor, communication skills are of paramount importance, and for these to be evident there has to be an inclination to engage with your patient.

The most likely place for specific questions to come up is in the oral, but once you are familiar with the different models, you could use the frameworks to help structure your written paper answers. However, in the orals, the examiners must get rather tired of people reciting Neighbour and Pendleton, so try and be a little more rounded in your approach (although well done for remembering these two).

What I have tried to do in this section is give a brief summary of several models. Of course, this is no substitute for reading the original texts from cover to cover, but it is probably a little easier to digest at this stage.

It is worth noting that the formal history-taking part of clinical management, if used prematurely, can stifle the patient's agenda. A patient's initial narrative is an important part of the consultation. It has been proved, contrary to popular belief, that the majority of patients will not go on to talk indefinitely, but will usually stop within 1 minute. Allowing patients to get their problem off their chest uninterrupted greatly increases satisfaction on all sides.

Everything you were afraid to ask about communication skills
Br J Gen Pract 2005; 55: 40–6

This discussion paper, by Skelton, starts by citing the Toronto consensus statement on communication: 'effective communication ... is a central clinical function which largely determines the patient's satisfaction and compliance and positively influences health outcomes'. It looks at the teaching of communication skills and their place in the curriculum, posing the philosophical question that rather than teaching communication skills, perhaps the focus should be on attitudes, in the belief that it would generate the appropriate communication skills.

Reflections on the doctor–patient relationship: from evidence to experience (MacKenzie lecture)
Br J Gen Pract 2005; 55: 793–801

Moira Stewart considers general practice to be 'whole-person medical practice' and gives this lecture with the understanding that doctor–patient relationships evolve over time and with shared experiences (with a common goal of diagnosis and cure). The six interactive components of the patient-centred methods discussed are summarised below:

- exploring disease and the patient's illness experience

- understanding the whole person

- finding common ground

- incorporating prevention and health promotion

- enhancing the patient–doctor relationship
- being realistic.

The paper concludes that without general practice there would be more confusion, fear and doubt.

Getting it right in the consultation: Hippocrates' problem; Aristotle's answer Dr John Gillies, Occasional Paper 86, The Royal College of General Practitioners

This paper considers many thoughts and approaches to medicine, decision making, ethical values and philosophies that have developed, mainly over the past 50 years, but drawing on work up to 2,000 years old (given the understanding that human nature has changed little over that time). Among others, Gillies considers Toon's analyses of several models of general practice, and McWhinney's (1996) description of the four main ways general practice differs from other specialties. These can be summarised as follows.

- General practice defines itself in terms of relationships, especially the doctor–patient relationship.
- We tend to think in terms of individuals rather than generalise.
- We have an organismic (i.e. consider the whole) rather than a mechanistic (i.e. the part) approach.
- It is the only major field that transcends the division between mind and body.

This will in no way be a quick read, but it would be worthwhile.

Balint model

This is a psychological model of the doctor–patient relationship. The understanding that doctors have feelings, and that these have a function within the consultation, form part of the model.

Balint explains that a patient's problem will have psychological and physical components, and that these will be interlinked. Indeed psychological problems may manifest themselves clinically. Individual doctors vary in their awareness of these points, but they can be trained to be more sensitive and aware.

Important features of the Balint model include the following:

- the doctor as a drug
- the child of a patient may be brought with a trivial problem for the patient to make contact (i.e. the child as the presenting complaint)
- elimination by appropriate examination
- collusion of anonymity
- 'The Flash'.

Berne's transactional analysis

Berne (1968) *The Games People Play*. Penguin Books, London

This model looks at the roles that patients and doctors take within the consultation, and identifies three 'ego' states:

- parent – critical or caring
- adult – logical
- child – dependent.

This is a useful model for analysing why consultations go wrong. Often a doctor will flit between adult and parent state, and the patient will flit between adult and child (and parent to a lesser degree). Imagine a consultation in which both the doctor and the patient assumed the role of 'child'. I'm sure you would agree that it is likely to be dysfunctional.

Stott and Davis model

This is a four-part model, and is probably the way that many of us deal with a consultation, certainly on the face of it.

Management of presenting problem	Management of continuing problem
Modification of health-seeking behaviour	Opportunistic health promotion

Neighbour's model: the inner consultation

This is a popular 'check point' model. It consists of the following steps.

1 *Connecting* – establishing a relationship; this needs rapport-building skills.

2 *Summarising* – 'What I am hearing is ...'; this needs the ability to listen and the skills to facilitate effective assessment.

3 *Hand over* – responsibility is given to the patient; this needs good communication skills to hand over the responsibility for management, because it involves negotiating and influencing (to a certain extent).

4 *Safety netting* – 'Have I missed anything?' and instructions for follow-up if ...; this needs predictive skills to suggest contingency plans for the worst-case scenario.

5 *House keeping* – 'Am I fit for the next patient?'; this needs self-awareness and the ability to file one consultation so that there is no effect on the next.

Pendleton model

This is otherwise known as the *social skills model*. It has seven tasks.

1 Define the reason for the patient's attendance, including the following:
   - the nature and history of the problems
   - their aetiology
   - the patient's ideas, concerns and expectations
   - the effects of the problems.
2 Consider other problems:
   - continuing other problems
   - at-risk factors.
3 Choose with the patient an appropriate action for each problem.
4 Achieve a shared understanding of the problems with the patient.
5 Involve the patient in the management of their case, and involve them in acceptance of appropriate responsibility for it.
6 Use time and resources appropriately.
7 Establish or maintain a relationship with the patient which helps in the achievement of other tasks.

Byrne and Long model

This is a six-point 'time sequence model' (i.e. it is based on the observed sequence of events).

1 The doctor establishes a relationship with the patient.
2 The doctor attempts to discover the patient's reason for attendance.
3 The doctor conducts a verbal (and physical) examination.
4 The doctor (with or without the patient) considers the problems.
5 The doctor (with or without the patient) makes a further plan (e.g. investigation, treatment, etc.).
6 Consultation is terminated, usually by the doctor.

Middleton agenda model

This is a four-point dynamic model in which the patient's agenda is paramount. It is not task orientated.

1 *Patient's agenda* – this includes the ideas and reasoning that underlie the problems presented.
2 *Doctor's agenda* – this includes risk factors, continuing problems, public health agenda, partnerships and personal agendas.

3 *Communication skills* – these can be chosen to reconcile the agendas (e.g. facilitation and negotiation).

4 *Negotiated plan* – this includes management of problems and health promotion.

Tiraxial model

This looks at the patient's problems in physical, psychological and social terms.

Heron model

This is a six-category intervention model, i.e. the doctor can use any of six types of intervention.

1 *Prescriptive* – instructions given.

2 *Informative* – explanations given.

3 *Confronting* – challenging but caring (e.g. on behaviour/presentation).

4 *Cathartic* – aids release of emotions (e.g. anger, laughter, tears).

5 *Catalytic* – encourages the patient's exploration of their feelings, thoughts and behaviour.

6 *Supportive* – of the problems and the solutions presented.

Calgary–Cambridge guide

This model can be summarised as follows:

1 *Initiating the session*:
 ● establishing a rapport
 ● identifying reasons for consultation.

2 *Gathering information*:
 ● exploration of the problem
 ● understanding the patient's perspective
 ● providing structure for the consultation.

3 *Building the relationship*:
 ● providing the correct amount and type of information
 ● aiding accurate recall and understanding
 ● achieving a shared understanding
 ● shared decision making
 ● negotiating a management plan.

4 *Closing the session*:
 ● final summary.

5 *Contracting* – establish a plan/contract with the patient.

6 *Safety netting* – similar to Neighbour's model.

7 *Final check* – before moving on.

Communicating risk to patients

We communicate levels of risk to patients and colleagues throughout most of our working day, for example in prescribing medication, explaining side effects, consenting a patient for a procedure, etc. The words we use to describe risk affect perception, which in turn may affect compliance with treatment, which in turn may affect success of a treatment and outcome.

Interpretation in words or figures:

Verbal	Frequency	Probability
Very common	>10%	>1 in 10
Common	1–10%	1 in 100 to 1 in 10
Uncommon	0.1–1%	1 in 1,000 to 1 in 100
Rare	0.01–0.1%	1 in 10,000 to 1 in 1,000

The British Heart Foundation (www.bhf.org.uk/factfiles) discussed various aspects that help in explaining risk to patients (**Factfile April 2005**). It makes the valid point that a patient's perception of risk is often very different from that of the health professional explaining the risk. Health professionals who have been trained in using decision aids (e.g. statistical aids such as percentages or probabilities, or visual aids) are able to change the context of their consultation.

Supporting decision making can involve several stages.

1 Clarifying the decision by explaining the problem.

2 Discussing the evidence base.

3 Acknowledging the patient's role in decision making.

4 Describing benefit and harm (avoid probabilities and try to use absolute, rather than relative, risk).

5 Understanding the patient's attitudes to the benefits described.

6 Considering how important the treatment is to the patient, and how confident they are in making the decision.

Shared decision making and risk communicating in practice
Br J Gen Pract 2004; 55: 6–13

This qualitative paper interviewed 20 clinicians skilled in shared decision making. It found that professionals respected patient involvement in decision making, and that decision-making skills to empower patients could be improved by addressing how consultations were scheduled in primary care, and raising patients' expectations for involvement.

Critical reading

At the risk of sounding like a secondary-school teacher, your ability to assess the quality of the work published will only improve if you practise. If you decide to take the MRCGP, usually three of the questions in the written paper are on critical appraisal. These seem to take more time to answer than candidates appreciate, which brings us back to the issue of practice.

It is useful to have a simple critical appraisal template that you can apply in order to structure the way you read and then apply to your answers. I have provided some examples of different methods you can try.

READER: an acronym to aid critical reading by general practitioners
Br J Gen Pract **1994; 44: 83–5**

R   Relevance:
  - to general practice
  - to your environment
  - general awareness.

E   Education:
  - behaviour modification
  - challenges to practices and beliefs.

A   Applicability:
  - own environment
  - generalisability.

D   Discrimination:
  - quality of the study
  - type of study: descriptive/randomised controlled trial
  - sample size
  - selection
  - controls
  - bias
  - results
  - statistics
  - conclusions.

E   Evaluation:
  - reflection.

R   Reaction:
  - implementation.

Remember, always try and be positive about a study first.

Template for critical appraisal

1 *Summary*
 – Concise statement of topic and conclusions.

2 *Introduction*
 – Is there a clear outline?

3 *Methods and design*
 – Are the selection and sample size appropriate?
 – What are the strengths and limitations?

4 *Results*
 – Is presentation clear?
 – Are results both clinically and statistically significant?

5 *Discussion*
 – Are statements true?

Keele University model

This method will help you to obtain the important information from each section (i.e. summarise the paper). This provides the basis for evaluating it.

1 *Is it of interest?*
 – Look at the abstract, title, authors etc.

2 *Motivation, why was it done?*
 – Look at the introduction, is it clear?
 – Who funded the research?

3 *Design: how was it done?*
 – Look at the methods: sample, recruitment, numbers, collection of data.
 – Measurements: are they valid/reliable?
 – Analysis: what statistics were used?
 – Any ethical problems or bias?

4 *Results: what did it find?*
 – Look at the results: are the data described and do the numbers add up?
 – Was statistical significance assessed?
 – Were all the data used?

5 *Conclusions: what are the implications?*
 – Look at the discussion.
 – Has anything been overlooked?
 – Are the findings relevant?

6 *Anything else of interest?*
 – For example, references.

Appraisal of a paper

1 Is the hypothesis clearly described?

2 Are the outcomes measured clearly described? If these are first mentioned in the results section, then the answer to this is no.

3 Are the characteristics of groups (e.g. inclusion/exclusion criteria) clearly described?

4 Are the interventions clearly described?

5 Are the main findings clearly described?

6 Does the study provide estimates of random variability in the data for the main outcomes?
   - If the data are non-normally distributed, the inter-quartile range should be quoted.
   - If the data are normally distributed, the standard error of the mean, standard deviation and confidence intervals should be used.

7 Have important adverse events been reported?

8 Have the characteristics of patients lost to follow-up been reported?

9 Have actual probability values been reported (e.g. $p = 0.04$ rather than $p < 0.05$)?

External validity

10 Were the subjects representative of the population?

11 Were the staff and facilities representative of the treatment that the majority of patients would receive?

Internal validity, bias (think selection and information)

12 Was the study blinded?

13 Were the statistical tests used appropriate (e.g. non-parametric tests should be used for data that are not normally distributed)?

14 Was compliance with the intervention reliable?

15 Were the main outcome measurements that were used reliable?

Implications of the study (the final part of appraisal of a paper)

16 What is the general importance in light of other research?

17 Can you extrapolate from the study group to general practice?

18 Is the size of the result observed important? The answer may be no, even if the results are statistically significant.

19 If you conclude that the results are important, what are their implications?
  • For patients?
  • For GPs?
    − workload
    − financially
    − education
    − resources
    − other members of the primary healthcare team.
  • Wider issues: ethics, right to choose.

Qualitative research

The approach is similar to quantitative appraisal.

• Focus on methods (e.g. interview techniques and settings) (source of internal bias), as well as the role of the researcher and their qualifications.

• Look at the quality-control measures used (e.g. content analysis, grounded theory).

• In qualitative research, the conclusions and discussions are not usually separate.

Statistics

Statistics is about gathering, communicating, analysing and interpreting information. In medical statistics we tend to use *inferential statistics*, in that we draw conclusions from a sample that has been drawn from the population.

When critiquing papers, or embarking on research or audit yourself, you need to have a fundamental understanding of the basics. I shall attempt to put the theory in simple terms and explain things which may otherwise be somewhat unclear. It is then a matter of actually reading the statistical analyses in papers to gain further understanding.

There are two distinct types of data.

1 *Qualitative data* − descriptive information.

2 *Quantitative data* − numerical information.

Quantitative data can be either *continuous* (e.g. 0.1 kg to 44 kg, all values within the span are possible), or they can be *discrete*, usually obtained by counting (e.g. 0, 1, 2, 3 ..., such as the number of moles present on the skin or shoe size).

Bar charts

A bar chart is a graphical representation of values/numbers.

• The height of the column is proportional to the frequency it represents.

• Each column should have the same width.

An example of a bar chart is shown below. There is obviously too little information on the axes for the chart to be useful!

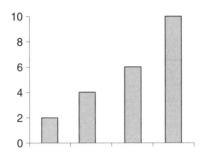

The number of packets of gum consumed per month.

Pie chart/pie diagram

This is a circle divided into sectors at angles that are proportional to the frequency of the data they represent. An example is shown below.

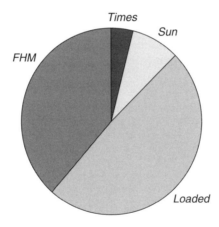

The number of times violence appeared in print.

Measures of location

Mode

This is the most commonly occurring value. It assumes that the modal class is divided into the same ratio.

The mode is time 20–29.9 minutes, *not* 60–120 minutes, as this modal class is longer (*see* table opposite).

It is possible to have more than one modal class.

Time taken to critique a paper (minutes)	Number of people
0–9.9	4
10–19.9	7
20–29.9	9
30–39.9	6
40–49.9	5
50–59.9	3
60–120	9

Median

This is the middle value of data once they have been placed in numerical order.
    For example: 3 4 5 6 7 **7** 8 8 8 10 15

The 7 in bold typeface is the median
    Or: 0 1 2 4 5 5 6 7

The median is halfway between 4 and 5, so is 4.5.

Mean

This generally means the average.

$$\text{Mean} = \frac{\text{sum of the values}}{\text{number of values}}$$

The mean and median are a measure of symmetry or lack of it.
    In a normal (Gaussian) distribution, the mode, median and mean all have the same value.

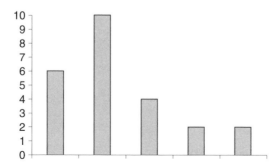

Positive skew.

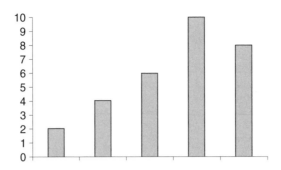

Negative skew.

Measures of dispersion

Range

This is the difference between extremes (i.e. the largest and the smallest). It does not take into account anything about the distribution of the data.

Quartile spread

- The median is halfway through the data.
- The point halfway between the lower extreme and the median is the *lower quartile*.
- The point halfway between the median and the upper extreme is the *upper quartile*.
- The difference between the upper and lower quartiles is the *interquartile range*.

Standard deviation

- Whereas range and interquartile range relate to the median, standard deviation relates to the spread about the mean.
- The standard deviation uses all values, and is therefore sensitive to outliers (i.e. extreme values).

SD = square root of the variance.

$$\text{Variance} = \frac{\text{sum of the square deviations from the mean}}{n}$$

In a normal distribution:

- 65% of values lie within 1 SD
- 95% of values lie within 2 SD
- 99% of values lie within 3 SD.

Probability

This indicates the degree of likelihood of an event happening, or the uncertainty of an event occurring.

$$\text{Probability of an outcome} = \frac{\text{number of events in the outcome}}{\text{total number of possible events}}$$

For example:

- the probability of rolling a 6 when throwing a dice is 1/6
- the probability of throwing a 6 followed by another 6 is $1/6 \times 1/6 = 1/36$ (i.e. probability of a *and* b, so multiply)
- the probability of throwing a 6 or a 4 is $1/6 + 1/6 = 2/6 = 1/3$ (i.e. probability of a *or* b, so add).

Errors

There are two types of error.

1 In *random error*, the sample mean deviates from the true mean despite the sample being representative.

2 In *systematic error*, the sample is not representative (i.e. there is bias).

Hypothesis test and p-value

This is a test of significance.

1 The first step is the statement of the null hypothesis: 'there is no difference between the two groups under study' (i.e. postulate the hypothesise that the intervention will have no effect).

2 The second step is to conduct a test of statistical significance based on the null hypothesis:
   - *t*-test
   - Chi-squared test.

3 The third step is the production of a *p*-value from the statistical tests.

The *p*-value is the probability of the result occurring by chance if the null hypothesis was true. If the *p*-value is small, then it is unlikely to have occurred by chance (i.e. it is a significant result). Usually $p < 0.05$ indicates a significant result. If $p < 0.01$, the result is highly significant (i.e. likely to have occurred by chance in <1% of cases).

It is important to appraise a study before taking the *p*-values as meaningful, because they may be irrelevant in the following circumstances:

- poor design of trial
- bias
- trial affected by confounding factors.

If there is a small sample size, then the statistical analysis may be unable to detect a significant difference when there may be one. This is referred to as the power of the study.

Confidence intervals

Confidence intervals (CI) are another way of assessing the effects of chance (c.f. *p*-value). They are a way of communicating the level of uncertainty, and they can be calculated for various statistical analyses (e.g. odds ratios, relative risks, risk difference, sensitivity, specificity, etc.).

- There is an upper and a lower value and, assuming the study was not biased, the true value can be expected to lie between these two values.
- Most studies use 95% CI or 95% confidence limits. This is usually two standard deviations either side of the mean.
- The wider the range of the CI, the less certain/significant the results are. The more people there are in the study, the smaller the interval will be.
- If the CI range includes zero, the result is not statistically significant.
- If the results are expressed as a ratio, then a CI including 1 is not statistically significant.
- The results are visual.

Risk

Measures of risk

New cases = incidence

Existing cases = prevalence

$$\text{Incidence} = \frac{\text{new illness episodes}}{\text{population at risk during a specific period of time}} \times 10^a$$

$$\text{Prevalence} = \frac{\text{number of individuals with existing disease}}{\text{population size during specific time period}} \times 100\%$$

Measures of association

Risk is calculated by comparing what happens to different groups of people. Consider a population that has been split into two subpopulations.

- Population 1 = population exposed to risk factor.
- Population 2 = population not exposed to risk factor.

Both populations have an associated risk of disease.

$$\text{Probability of disease/death} = \text{Risk (R)} = \frac{\text{number with the disease}}{\text{number at risk of the disease}} = \frac{d}{n}$$

$$\text{Risk difference (RD)} = \text{Risk 1} - \text{Risk 2} = \frac{d_1}{n_1} - \frac{d_2}{n_2}$$

$$\text{Relative risk (RR)} = \frac{R_1}{R_2} = \frac{d_1/n_1}{d_2/n_2} = \frac{d_1 \times n_2}{d_2 \times n_1}$$

$$\text{Absolute risk (AR)} = \frac{R_1 - R_2}{R_1}$$

Absolute risk and relative risk are figures used to assess the strength of a relationship between a disease and any factor that might affect it.

Absolute risk (AR)

$$= \frac{\text{the number of events that occur in the treated and control group}}{\text{number of people in that group}}$$

The absolute risk reduction is the difference between the control group and the treated group.

$$\text{ARR} = \text{ARC} - \text{ART}$$

Relative risk (or *risk ratio*) in randomised controlled trials and cohort studies, or relative odds in cohort or case controlled studies, is the ratio of absolute risks of the disease between the two groups.

- If $RR < 1$, then intervention reduces the risk of the outcome being studied.
- If $RR = 1$, then the treatment has no effect on the outcome being studied.
- If $RR > 1$, then the intervention increases the risk of the outcome being studied.

Odds

Odds are a way of representing probability. They are defined as the ratio of the probability of an event happening to that of it not happening (i.e. risk).

Odds ratio

This is a measure of the effectiveness of a treatment. It is an estimate of relative risk.

$$\text{Odds ratio} = \frac{\text{Odds in the treated group}}{\text{Odds in the control group}}$$

- If OR < 1, the effects of the treatment are less than those of the control treatment.
- If OR $= 1$, the effects of the treatment are no different from the control treatment.
- If OR > 1, the effects of the treatment are greater than the control treatment.

The effects can be good or bad.

Diagnostic testing

	Disease positive	Disease negative	Total
Test positive	a	b	a + b
Test negative	c	d	c + d
Total	a + c	b + d	a + b + c + d

$$\text{Sensitivity} = \frac{\text{Number of test positive and disease positive}}{\text{Number of disease positive}} = \frac{a}{a + c}$$

$$\text{Specificity} = \frac{\text{Number of test negative and disease negative}}{\text{Number of disease negative}} = \frac{d}{b + d}$$

Positive predictive value = the probability that an individual diagnosed test positive will be true positive

$$= \frac{a}{a + b}$$

Negative predictive value = probability that an individual diagnosed test negative will be a true negative

$$= \frac{d}{c + d}$$

Number needed to treat (NNT)

This is the number of people you would need to treat with a specific intervention (e.g. aspirin for people having a heart attack) to see one occurrence of a specific outcome (e.g. prevention of death).

$$\text{NNT} = \frac{1}{\text{Absolute risk reduction}}$$

This value can be multiplied by 100 if using a percentage.
Thus, the smaller the absolute risk reduction, the higher the NNT.

The number needed to screen – an adaptation of the number needed to treat
Journal of Medical Screening **2001; 8: 114–15**

This paper suggests that estimates of NNT should carry a health warning. The concept of preventing one event should be compared with the more likely probability that several people benefit by having an event delayed by a few years. For example an antihypertensive drug that reduces the incidence of stroke by 30% can be interpreted in two ways: the drug prevented 30% of strokes (with no effect on the other 70%); or that all strokes in the treatment group were delayed by 3 years.

Other statistical terms

Bias

This is the deviation of the results from the truth – a one sided inclination of the mind.

- *Publication bias* occurs where studies with positive results are more likely to be published.

- *Selection bias* occurs where there are systematic differences between sample and target populations.

- *Information bias* occurs where there are systematic errors in measurement of outcome or exposure.

Heterogeneity

This term is used when there is no overlap of the trials used in a meta-analysis.

Homogeneity 'similarity'

This term is used to state that all trials on the plot have an overlap of confidence intervals (i.e. in a meta-analysis).

Meta-analysis

This is a paper that looks at a number of original research papers in an attempt to answer a question by summarising several papers. The methodology of the search (i.e. not confined to English, using more than one search engine, including unpublished trials) is a good indicator of the validity of the results.

Validity

This refers to how rigorous a study is.

- *Study validity* is the validity with respect to internal and external bias.

- *Internal validity* is the degree to which conclusions internal to the study are legitimate.

- *External validity* is the degree to which conclusions generated from the sample could be generalised to the target population.

Study designs

Experimental study designs
- *Randomised controlled trials* — a minimum of two groups to which patient allocation is random, where one of the groups is the control (i.e. non-experimental group).

Observational study designs
- *Cross-sectional survey* — a study in which the sample frame is observed at one particular time. It gives prevalence estimates, and cause and effect are difficult to establish.

- *Cohort study* — a longitudinal follow-up of two or more cohorts (groups) with recorded exposure to a risk factor. It provides comparative incidence estimates between exposed and non-exposed groups. There can be surveillance bias.

- *Case-controlled study* — this is used to compare two groups when prevalence is low. Odds ratios are used for analysis.

Forest plot

This is a pictorial representation of odds ratios in the form of horizontal lines. They represent the 95% CI of each trial, with a vertical line representing the point where the study intervention would have no effect (i.e. if the horizontal line crosses the vertical line then the result is not significant).

Funnel plot

This is a graph in which each study is represented by a dot, the position of which depends on the size of the effect of the intervention (on the horizontal axis) and the size of the study (on the vertical axis).

Part 3

Introduction

Part 3 is all about the final hurdle – the exam. The MRCGP exam tests an incredible range of knowledge, clinical and communication skills, as well as professional attitudes (a key point to remember is that whatever your personal feelings and beliefs, you are taking this exam in a professional capacity).

It is important to read and understand the current regulations for each module at the time of application (www.rcgp.org.uk). The current exam will be replaced by the new examination, to be called the nMRCGP – this should be implemented by 2008. There is a syllabus published on the website. It should be considered essential reading, and can be used as a check list. It is described as a guide, and it by no means includes everything. The syllabus discusses the General Medical Council's *Good Medical Practice* (2001) document and the different areas as they are likely to appear in the exam:

- good clinical care
- maintaining good medical practice
- relationships with patients
- working with colleagues
- teaching, training, assessment and appraisal
- probity
- health and performance of other doctors.

When you are working for the exams, I would encourage you to consider topics in isolation (either individually, in a study group – this might help you to focus on the work and would be a good forum for discussions – or with work colleagues) before you think about looking at exam papers. As the exam approaches, try working the sample papers (against the clock is a must for at least one of the papers). The answers given here for the written and oral examinations are suggestions of what would be important to include. They are comprehensive but not exhaustive. There will be points you feel should have been included – so include them, this is your exam. Depending on how strongly you feel, please email suggestions to me at gear@doctors.org.uk.

Multiple-choice questions for the MRCGP

These papers are machine marked, and they test a huge amount of knowledge in a relatively short period of time. The papers will include: medicine, management, administration issues, research, epidemiology and statistics. For this reason it is not advisable to sit the exam until you have done at least 3 months of general practice.

When you are revising, remember that ENT, ophthalmology, dermatology, etc., will feature in the exam.

The way to improve at multiple-choice question (MCQ) exams is to do sample questions, mark them, and read around the questions you got wrong *and* the questions you got right. This will expand your knowledge base – especially if some of your right answers were lucky guesses.

In the MRCGP exam, do not be surprised at the number of extended matching questions (EMQs) on the paper. There will be instructions for particular questions, and usually you have to choose the single best answer for the stem question asked, but do not assume that this is the case. Another favourite is to have an abstract supplied with key words missing, which you then have to identify correctly from a list. Again the exam information will go through different question styles and give examples. On the day, make sure you read the information given and the questions very carefully.

For MCQ exams, it is important to know how to interpret certain phrases. The following definitions are from the college guidelines, but you will find almost identical definitions in most MCQ books.

- *Diagnostic, characteristic, pathognomonic* or *in the vast majority* – implies that the feature would occur in 90% of cases.

- *Typically, frequently, significantly, commonly* or *in a substantial majority* – implies that the feature would occur in 60% of cases or more.

- *In the majority* – implies that the feature would occur in 50% of cases or more.

- *In the minority* – implies that the feature would occur in less than 50% of cases.

- *Low chance* or *in a substantial minority* – implies that a feature may occur in up to 30% of cases.

- *Has been shown, recognised* or *reported* – all refer to evidence found in authoritative medical texts.

Here I have included some samples of my own MCQs. I have not produced a paper as such, for reasons of space. There are many MCQ and EMQ books available (e.g. *EMQs for the MRCGP Paper 2* by Hayley Dawson and Anna Trigell, 2005; Radcliffe Publishing).

Sample multiple-choice questions

Questions

Answer True or False for each of the following.

Dermatological emergencies include:

1 erythrasma
2 erythrodermic psoriasis
3 epidermal necrolysis
4 Norwegian scabies
5 pitted keratolysis.

Diseases that are known to koebnerise include:

6 pityriasis rosea
7 psoriasis
8 lichen sclerosis
9 lichen planus
10 erythema multiforme
11 pityriasis lichenoides.

The eye drops below are noted for the following:

12 bradycardia with pilocarpine
13 cyclopentolate can precipitate glaucoma
14 when using atropine drops for refraction, the effects can last up to 2 months
15 exacerbation of asthma with timolol
16 Rose Bengal is useful for visualising corneal ulceration.

The following are recognised as improving survival rates in acute myocardial infarction:

17 aspirin
18 thrombolysis given within 48 hours of onset of the pain
19 atenolol
20 nifedipine
21 immediate percutaneous transluminal angioplasty
22 warfarin.

In drug treatment of non-insulin dependent diabetes mellitus:

23 sulphonylureas suppress appetite
24 metformin may cause hypoglycaemia
25 chlorpropramide is a suitable sulphonylurea to use in the elderly
26 thiazolidindiones are associated with liver damage
27 prandial glucose regulators are not yet licensed in the UK.

With regard to postnatal depression:

28 1 in 50 women become depressed after childbirth
29 the Edinburgh postnatal depression scale is designed for use 6–8 weeks post-natally
30 postnatal depression commonly starts 3–5 days after childbirth
31 SSRIs are of proven benefit.

In the diagnosis of altered bowel habit
For each patient in questions 32 to 36, select the most likely cause of the problem from the list of options below.

a carcinoma of the colon
b irritable bowel syndrome

c *Campylobacter* enteritis
d giardiasis
e Crohn's disease
f ischaemic colitis
g pseudomembranous colitis
h laxative abuse
i chronic pancreatitis

32 An 18-year-old girl has been amenorrhoeic for 6 months, has lost a lot of weight and has developed loose stools (at least four times a day).

33 A 28-year-old female patient has recently been made redundant. She has started with episodic diarrhoea with small-volume stools and a feeling of incomplete defecation. There is abdominal pain and bloating.

34 A 22-year-old student has returned from Russia with episodic loose stool and is passing offensive wind.

35 A 48-year-old man with a family history of polyposis coli defaulted from the surveillance programme some years ago. Over the past 3 months he has developed altered bowel habit and has lost a little weight. There has been one episode of rectal bleeding.

36 A 36-year-old businessman has completed a 2-week course of cephalexin. He has now developed a fever, diarrhoea and cramping abdominal pains.

For each of the drugs in questions 37 to 41, choose the most appropriate side effect from the list of options below.

a oligogyric crisis
b serotonin syndrome
c exfoliative dermatitis
d venous thrombosis
e bradycardia
f hypertension
g dry mouth

37 Tamoxifen.
38 Atenolol.
39 Tolterodine (Detrusitol).
40 Fluoxetine.
41 Metoclopramide.

For each of questions 42 to 48, choose the most appropriate item from the list of options below.

a no precautions needed
b 7
c 14

d 5
e 19
f 21
g 3

42 A patient needing postcoital contraception has presented too late for Levonelle-2. If she has a regular 28-day cycle, up to what day is it acceptable to use an IUD?

43 Microval (a progestogen-only contraceptive) is started on day 1 of your patient's period. For how many days should she use additional contraception?

44 A patient is 4 hours late taking her Loestrin-20 contraceptive pill. How many days extra precautions are required?

45 Your patient is changing from a combined contraceptive pill to Noriday, without a break between pill packs. For how many days are extra precautions required?

46 Your patient is breastfeeding and needs contraception. How many days post-partum can the progestogen-only pill Femulen be started?

47 If your post-partum patient wanted to start Micronor (her usual progestogen-only pill), when could this be started from?

48 Within how many days of unprotected sexual intercourse should Levonelle-2 be taken to be effective as postcoital contraception?

The Mental Health Act
For each of the statements in questions 49 to 55, choose the most appropriate section from the list of options below.

a Section 2
b Section 3
c Section 4
d Section 5
e Section 7
f Section 12
g Section 135
h Section 136

49 This is used for the assessment of a patient for up to 28 days.

50 This is used only in an emergency.

51 This can be used by the police to detain a person they believe is suffering from a mental illness.

52 This is used for compulsory treatment of a patient with an established diagnosis.

53 This is appropriate for guardianship.

54 This gives the police right of entry into private premises to remove a patient to a place of safety.

55 This is used to approve doctors who are recognised as having specialised expertise in mental health.

Medical statistics

Match each of the statements in questions 56 to 60 with the most appropriate term from the list of options below.

a correlation
b confidence
c incidence
d predictive value
e confounding

56 This depends on the sensitivity and specificity of a test.

57 This needs to be eliminated in a reliable study.

58 This depends on the prevalence of a disease in the population studied.

59 This is the occurrence of new cases in a population over a given period of time.

60 This occurs when a variable changes in a way that directly relates to another variable.

Hypertension screening

	Screening test positive	Screening test negative
Hypertension present	340	51
Hypertension not present	82	172

For each of the items in questions 61 to 65, select the most appropriate answer from the list of options below.

a 51/391
b 51/223
c 340/391
d 340/42251
e 82/25482
f 82/422
g 172/223
h 172/254
i 340
j 51
k 82
l 172

61 Specificity.

62 Sensitivity.

63 Positive predictive value.

64 Negative predictive value.

65 False negative.

Hip screening test performed in neonates

	Screening test positive	Screening test negative
Problem present	29	42
Problem not present	64	364

For each of the items in questions 66 to 70, choose the most appropriate answer from the list of options below.

a 29/93
b 29/71
c 42/71
d 42/408
e 64/93
f 64/428
g 364/406
h 364/428
i 29
j 42
k 64
l 364

66 Positive predictive value.

67 Negative predictive value.

68 Specificity.

69 Sensitivity.

70 False negative.

Answers

1 False
2 True
3 True
4 False
5 False

6 False

7 True

8 True

9 True

10 True

11 False

12 False (seen with beta-blocker drops)

13 True (it is mydriatic)

14 False (2 weeks)

15 True

16 True

17 True

18 False (needs to be within 24 hours)

19 True (ISIS 1)

20 False

21 False (significant mortality)

22 False

23 False (they stimulate insulin secretion, so stimulate appetite)

24 False (sulphonylureas do)

25 False (this has the longest half-life; tolbutamide would be a better option)

26 True (troglitazone was withdrawn because of this)

27 False

28 False (1 in 10)

29 True

30 False (commonly 4–6 weeks; baby blues 3–5 days)

31 True (as are tricyclic antidepressants)

32 h

33 b

34 d

35 a

36 g

37 d

38 e

39 h

40 b

41 a

42 e

43 c

44 a

45 a

46 b
47 f
48 g

49 a
50 c
51 h
52 b
53 e
54 g
55 f

56 d
57 e
58 d
59 c
60 a

61 h
62 c
63 d
64 g
65 j

66 a
67 g
68 h
69 b
70 j

The written paper

The main aim of the written paper is to examine your ability to integrate and apply theoretical knowledge and professional values within the setting of primary healthcare in the UK.

The written paper is an arm cramping three and a half hours long, but not one person coming out of the exam has been heard to claim they had plenty of time. Make sure you have done at least one past paper against the clock to prepare yourself. Past papers can be downloaded from the college website, including the critical reading sections (www.rcgp.org.uk). Unfortunately, there are no model answers, just examiners' comments, but they are still a must, and the comments make clear the approach that you should take to score extra marks.

Excluding the critical reading questions, this paper is mainly about your ability to problem solve. As in real life, the most important aspect is not knowing all the answers but asking the right questions along the way, and taking the time to explore all the options.

The following suggestions might help you in preparing for the exam.

- Keep up to date. This goes for all areas of the exam as well as at work.
- Consider joining a study group. You can cover much more ground, and it helps to keep you motivated. Look at hot topics, GP issues, questions, etc.
- Practise against the clock, and try to stick to 15 minutes per question.
- Try to structure your answers rather than write freestyle. It will help you to think and the examiner to mark more quickly (so is less frustrating for them).
- Think broadly, and try to include ethical and cultural issues as well as personal development points.
- A course can be helpful, but it is not a necessity. Before you choose and pay for one, try to find people who have been on any of the ones you are considering, as some are better than others.

I have set out a 'paper', consisting of 12 questions (but no critical reading), all of which have either been real cases or arisen in practice.

In this section, I suggest that you give yourself a maximum of three hours (i.e. deduct the 30-minute reading time usually given for the critical reading). If at all possible try to treat it as a mock exam as this will get you used to formulating and writing your answers quickly. I have written a section on the process of critical reading and I really do advocate that you practise this on a regular basis (in both the journals and from the sample papers on the Royal College website) to improve both your skills and your speed. There are also several comprehensively written books on critical reading.

The answers are printed below the questions. It is all too easy to take a sneaky look at the answers, but then you will be left not knowing what you really do know and where your gaps are. Compare your answers with ours, and those of your colleagues, friends and even your trainer.

If you make it to the end (or get bored), then make up some of your own problem-based questions. Try keeping a list of problems or heartsinks from work. This may help you to understand the issues, and your heartsinks may become success stories. This is a method to take forward for your personal development plan. The exam is not about catching you out, but about testing your approach to real problems that you may encounter in everyday practice.

Written question 1

You are asked to take a call by your receptionist. A young mother is wanting advice about her 8-year-old son who has a cold and has developed a blotchy red rash. How do you deal with such a request?

This question is testing your approach to telephone consultations. This is an expanding role in general practice, and if handled incorrectly the consequences could be disastrous.

The telephone consultation lends itself to Neighbour's consultation model.

1 Introduce yourself.

2 Establish who you are speaking to and who is the patient.

3 Establish a rapport, do not rush. Actively listen and ask questions to clarify.

4 Summarise the problem or question.

5 Agree a plan.

6 Safety net (this is very important).

7 Make accurate records at the time, and do not forget to date and time the entry.

Practice points

- Triaging of calls, whose role should it be: receptionist, nurse, duty doctor?
  - what would be the safest method and make the best use of time?

- Role of the nurses:
  - is there a need for expansion of their role?
  - is there an individual wish for their roles to expand (to include nurse prescribing, for example)?

- Accessibility of the doctor:
  - for emergencies only or immediate access?
  - for enquiries (call back/telephone access), is it worth setting aside a set time of the day when patients know they can phone?
  - would increased accessibility improve patient satisfaction?

- Is there a need for protocols:
  - for access?
  - for triage?
  - for telephone consultations?

Doctor issues

- Duty to patients:
  - you should be accessible at a convenient time for them
  - if you are not happy with a clinical situation, do not compromise patient safety, but arrange to see the patient
  - medical point: is there a need to make a diagnosis and treat, determine what over-the-counter remedies, etc., have been tried?

- Workload:
  - telephone accessibility may reduce the number of appointments/home visits needed (i.e. could expand to include not just acute requests)
  - it may be time-consuming to get the notes, check the information, and ensure that the patient really does understand any issues you feel are important.

- Telephone consultation skills:
  - these need to be good (clear understanding, management plan, safety netting, etc.)
  - be fully aware of the risks of misunderstanding
  - increased patient and doctor satisfaction can result if it is done well.

- Learning needs:
  - develop consultation and communication skills
  - audit of outcomes (especially if expanding to include other areas such as asthma)
  - record keeping, etc.

- Stress:
  - this may increase (the paranoia of being wrong and missing a non-verbal clue or sign) as well as decrease (one less patient to see).

- Prescribing issues:
  - a multitude of issues are raised when you have not seen the patient. The same explanation of use, side effects, interactions, etc., should occur.

Patient issues

- Why are they phoning?
  - are there appointment problems, did they feel it too trivial to waste an appointment, has there been a similar family case that had more serious outcome, etc.?
- If they were phoning just for advice, are they aware of NHS Direct?

Other issues

- NHS Direct role:
  - advertise in surgery (advice line for minor illnesses).
- Pharmacists:
  - roles are expanding, especially in over-the-counter self-management.
- Public health:
  - advertising campaigns for self-management of minor self-limiting illnesses.
- Cultural and social factors (e.g. access to a telephone, language barriers, etc.).

Written question 2

How would you explain a diagnosis of IBS (irritable bowel syndrome) to a patient? You have made the diagnosis on history (ROME II criteria), normal examination and investigation.

Irritable bowel syndrome is the most common functional gastrointestinal problem seen in practice. There is no known cause, and it is likely to have a multi-factorial aetiology.

Common factors that can affect IBS are:

- diet, although not because of allergy

- stress (in more than 50% of patients)

- gastrointestinal infections (e.g. following *Campylobacter* infection).

The diagnosis would need to be discussed sensitively, rather than dismissively, given the probable degree of symptoms.

Give the patient a chance to ask questions – in particular to explore his or her own ideas and concerns.

How might IBS affect a patient's life?

These areas need to be considered individually.

- Pain:
  - this is mainly due to abdominal bloating and spasm, although haemorrhoids can develop secondary to straining
  - IBS patients tend to have a lower pain threshold (clinically proven in trials).

- Psychological:
  - anxiety or depression may be a trigger or a resultant factor
  - chronic pain is known to affect psychological morbidity.

- Work-related factors:
  - pain may impair performance or make work impossible (i.e. the disorder has socioeconomic implications).

- Family life:
  - if the pain and the unpredictability of the symptoms are long-standing, this may affect relationships (e.g. psychological aspects, dyspareunia, etc.).

What treatment has been proven to be of benefit?

IBS is difficult to treat. Several options found to be of help are listed below, although finding the one that is beneficial for your patient will probably be a case of trial and error. A large part of the treatment is explanation and reassurance. Consideration of dietary changes (including fibre content – both vegetable and whole grain) and increasing exercise is worthwhile.

- Antispasmodics:
  - mebeverine (NNT = 6) (inhibits intestinal smooth muscle contraction)
  - hyoscine (NNT = 9) (anticholinergic effects).

- Bulking agents:
  - ispaghula husk (NNT = 4).

- Anti-diarrhoeal agents:
  - loperamide (NNT = 3).

- Antidepressants (not for antidepressant effect):
  - low-dose tricyclics (NNT = 3)
  - $5HT_4$ agonists (improve constipation)
  - $5HT_3$ antagonists (reduce diarrhoea).

These figures have been taken from Primary Care Society for Gastroenterology guidelines.

- Complementary therapy:
  - hypnosis, cognitive behavioural therapy, biofeedback and psychotherapy have all been reported to be useful in certain cases
  - relaxation techniques, Chinese herbal medicine and acupuncture may also help, but as yet no convincing data have been published to support the claims.

When explaining the diagnosis it is important to discuss management options and develop a plan together with the patient.

Written question 3

You are given the role of improving diabetic care in your practice. How would you tackle the project?

It is known that lack of structure increases mortality in diabetic care, so organisation of services is of great importance.

With the publication of the Delivery Strategy for the National Service Framework for Diabetes and the implications of the new contract, this is an important area to have in order.

Determine the objectives

- Patient groups to be targeted:
  - NIDDM
  - IDDM
  - diet-controlled diabetes and impaired glucose tolerance
  - screening issues (e.g. in coronary heart disease groups).

- Look at the evidence base, new contract quality areas and Government guidelines on what the goals should be, especially with regard to the following:
  - blood pressure control (HOT study)
  - HBA_{1C} targets (UKPDS 33)
  - chiropody and ophthalmology checks
  - weight, obesity, diet and exercise
  - cholesterol and lipids.

Need to co-ordinate with secondary care where possible

Practice meeting to include all people to be involved clinically

- Develop objectives.

- Write guidelines or adopt previously written ones.

- Write leaflets or adopt previously written ones.

- Protocols, patient group directives and clinical management plans need to be written, depending on nurse involvement.

- Appointment system and clinic set-up (computer recall and template use for recall).

Audit current standards

- This should include a patient questionnaire on quality and satisfaction.

- Implement changes and set timescales.

- Re-audit (i.e. complete the audit cycle) after the implementation of the changes.

Significant event analysis

- Problems from clinic.

- Management points to be learned from mistakes.

Depending on your practice population, be aware of cultural issues and have appropriate advice to hand (e.g. Ramadan) in the most appropriate language.

Further issues

- Funding, equipment, register.

- Take into account the holistic, patient-centred approach, including some of the following issues:
  - flu and pneumococcal counselling
  - psychological impact of the disease
  - pre-conceptual counselling, etc.

If you were to develop the role of screening within your practice, what would be your rationale for including abdominal circumference measurement?

Although there is no formal screening programme for diabetes, many practices check a fasting glucose in patients with other cardiovascular morbidities, as well as in those with risk factors (such as a family history, obesity or gestational diabetes).

Historically, the body mass index has been used as a measure of obesity, but it is known that this can classify some patients as obese when in fact they are incredibly fit with a huge muscle mass, and it gives little idea as to the body fat content of an individual. Abdominal obesity is a known risk factor for cardiovascular disease, and although in diabetic and heart disease clinics patients are offered secondary prevention strategies to treatment, the abdominal girth (especially when someone is losing weight) would be a useful measurement in any clinic to monitor progress.

Currently, abdominal circumference is used as a ratio (waist–hip ratio) and forms part of the definition of the metabolic syndrome. The World Health Organization guidelines for diagnosing metabolic syndrome are as follows.

● Impaired fasting glucose or impaired glucose tolerance test, or diabetes, or insulin resistance plus one or more of the following:
  – waist–hip ratio >0.85 (in women) or >0.9 (in men), and/or a BMI >30 kg/m^2
  – triglycerides >1.7 mM and/or HDL-C <0.9 mM (women), <1.0 mM (men)
  – blood pressure >140/90 mmHg
  – microalbuminuria: urinary albumin excretion rate >20 μg/min.

However, there have been several studies that have looked at the use of waist–hip ratio as a measure for coronary heart disease risk as it seems to be more effective at predicting risk of myocardial infarction.

Obesity and the risk of myocardial infarction in 27,000 participants from 52 countries: a case-control study
Lancet **2005; 366: 1640–9**

This was a standardised case-control study of 27,098 (12,461 cases and 14,637 controls) participants (in 52 countries, representing several major ethnic minorities) which assessed the relation of BMI, waist and hip circumferences, and waist-to-hip ratio to myocardial infarction overall and for each group. The waist-to-hip ratio and waist and hip circumferences were closely ($p < 0.0001$) associated with risk of myocardial infarction, even after adjustment for other risk. The population-attributable risk of myocardial infarction for increased waist-to-hip ratio in the top two quintiles was 24.3% (95% CI 22.5–26.2) compared with only 7.7% (6.0–10.0) for the top two quintiles of BMI. The authors concluded that waist-to-hip ratio showed a graded and highly significant association with myocardial infarction risk worldwide, and recommended that there be a redefinition of obesity based on waist-to-hip ratio instead of BMI, as this would increase the estimate of myocardial infarction attributable to obesity in most ethnic groups.

Written question 4

You receive a health authority circular about a patient who is suspected of attempting to obtain drugs such as dihydrocodeine and temazepam under various different names, usually as a temporary resident. As you read through the circular it becomes increasingly apparent that you have probably seen the woman and issued her with the drugs. How would you deal with the situation?

Seeing temporary residents and issuing drugs for patients with whom you are not familiar is a relatively common scenario. Although it would have seemed the correct decision to prescribe the medication when you saw the patient, in this case it would appear someone is defrauding the system and putting herself, and maybe others, at risk.

Patient issues

- Why do the drugs need to be obtained deceitfully (i.e. what gains are in this for the patient)?
  - because of overuse or dependence?
  - for their retail value?
  - for another person who is dependent?

- Can she be contacted (has she given a fake address and telephone number) to exclude her from the enquiry, or to confirm her involvement?

- Is there any drug dependence or criminal history (i.e. is this a repeat offence or a new problem that is more amenable to help)?

- Psychological state – the patient will need a full assessment; are there other underlying medical or psychiatric problems?

Doctor issues

You need to be as certain as possible that this could be the same patient.

- Confidentiality:
  - you have a duty of care to this patient, even if she is a temporary resident who needs help
  - the GMC guidelines on confidentiality say that you can disclose information if the patient poses a serious risk to themself or others
  - disclose only what is necessary (e.g. you may not need to mention the medical reasons for requesting the treatment).

- Defence organisation – it is important, if you have any doubts, to discuss with your defence union what it would be prudent to disclose.

- Who to inform:
  - the health authority contact
  - the police who are dealing with the case
  - other partners and reception staff, in case of future attendance
  - other practices in the area if they have not received the circular.

- Written account:
  - it is important to keep your own written account for future reference
  - if this case ends up in court, you may be asked for more information than you put in your statement, and it would not be wise to rely on your memory.

- Personal development issues:
  - you need to be aware, and discuss if necessary, feelings of negativity and betrayal, etc.

  – were you singled out for any particular reason?
  – do you have a mentor or are you part of a Balint group where you may discuss
    the issues further?

Practice issues

- Temporary residents:
  – all forms should be fully completed
  – if NHS numbers, etc., are not known, should the patient's own GP be contacted
    for the information prior to the patient being seen?
  – should doctors repeat prescribe for temporary residents? This is not a simple 'yes
    or no' issue. Should certain drugs be excluded?
  – practice development issues (for example the circulation and storage of
    circulars).

- Computer/information technology:
  – all patients should be input so creating not only a trail but a complete record
    (especially important with plans for future sharing of electronic records).

- Use of the Internet to confirm GPs and address supplied:
  – www.gpinfo.com
  – www.streetmap.co.uk.

- Prescriptions:
  – no hand-written scripts if possible
  – if done through the computer this creates a log that is easier to audit.

- Significant event analysis:
  – is this a case that all the team could learn from?

- Consider audit:
  – on temporary residents
  – any repeat visits of temporary residents.

Written question 5

*In light of the strategy for sexual health, what implications would HIV testing have in
primary care?*

Approximately 30,000 people in the UK have HIV, and this number is still rising. The
sexual health strategy recommends that all GPs should offer HIV counselling and
testing. Currently less than 1% of practices offer this service (7% in London).

HIV is increasingly considered as a chronic, manageable problem. The current test is
HIV p24 antigen, and the HIV antibody test can be used to look for previous infection.

Routine screening in pregnancy is already offered in virtually all areas. This tends
to be blanket screening, rather than identifying the population at increased risk. It has
the obvious benefit that if the patient is HIV positive, and this is discovered before
the birth and early on in the pregnancy, it is possible to prevent/reduce transmission
to the foetus from 20–30% to 2%.

Doctor and practice issues

- Improved and extended service for patients.

- Improved communication (i.e. GPs are now more likely to be aware if their patients are on treatment for HIV, and can alter their other prescribing accordingly).

- Education and training (counselling skills, current treatment for HIV and AIDS, etc.):
  - what sort of advice to be giving (shaving, tooth brushing, what to do if the patient cuts themselves, etc.)
  - need to be aware of associated drug misuse and the implications of this for management and transmission of the disease
  - www.hiv-druginteractions.org is a dedicated website to check whether medication interacts with antiretrovirals.

- Workload implications:
  - time for screening and counselling
  - arranging for samples to be taken in an anonymous fashion if required
  - dealing with positive results (i.e. referral if necessary)
  - ensuring that repeat tests are carried out where necessary
  - other swabs that need doing or hepatitis B status (especially if it is late on Friday night and the patient is unlikely to return, which will mean swabs sitting around all weekend thus increasing the false negative rate)
  - contact tracing, and who will take the responsibility if the patient will not?
  - the RCGP has developed a Five ALHIVE guide for screening to encourage GPs to become involved.

- Confidentiality issues:
  - if samples are not labelled anonymously anyone can see the names. Should the issue be of any concern given that all of us working in the health service are bound by the same level of confidentiality?
  - if you have a positive result and the patient will not inform their partner(s) (especially if their partner is a patient of yours), where would your responsibilities lie and how would you deal with such conflict?

- Improved job satisfaction as skills and service develop.

- Resources:
  - GP, nurse and phlebotomy time
  - cost of the tests, administration and follow-up
  - if diagnosed early, morbidity and mortality can be dramatically decreased with treatment. This will mean higher drug costs for a longer period of time.
- Audit (i.e. appointment uptake/DNA rate for screening tests):
  - positive results (is screening being performed appropriately?)
  - outcome and patient satisfaction with an in-house service. Would patients self-select the relative anonymity of secondary care?

Primary healthcare team issues

- What would be their level of involvement in case selection, screening and contact tracing?

- Counselling following positive results.

- Dentist – again if positive, as only certain dentists will accept HIV-positive patients.

- Nurses – general all-round input, especially at the AIDS stage of the disease.

Patient issues

- Increased accessibility, and acceptance in normality, for requesting an HIV test for patients – general practice is generally much more accessible than secondary care.

- Increased patient satisfaction.

- Improved doctor–patient relationship because of GP involvement.

- Patient may lack confidence in:
  - GP knowledge as GPs are generalists not specialists
  - confidentiality within the practice (including bumping into acquaintances).

- Improved long-term outcome, i.e. reduction in mortality and morbidity.

- Improved quality of life.

Cultural and language barriers

- You need to consider patients' needs:
  - whether an interpreter need be employed – this has associated confidentiality issues
  - gender problems – a female may not consent to be seen by a male doctor, and vice versa, for swabs (as part of a thorough health screening in this scenario), etc.

Secondary care implications

- Would free up appointments for more complicated patients, so that GPs would be able to access secondary care more easily when a result is positive.

- Improved shared care and interprofessional relations.

- There may be a need for guidelines for HIV management and a shared-care approach (drawn up by both primary and secondary care physicians).

Written question 6

Margaret is a 66-year-old woman who had retired 18 months ago from running an excellent nursing home in the area. She was diagnosed shortly afterwards with ovarian cancer (for which she had nursed her sister). On seeing her today, despite morphine, her abdominal pain is becoming increasingly difficult to control. What can you do to help her?

The World Health Organization has defined palliative care as follows:

> The active total care of patients whose disease is not responsive to curative treatment. Control of pain, of other symptoms and of psychological, social and spiritual problems is paramount. The goal of palliative care is achievement of the best quality of life for patients and their families.

There is a lot to offer this woman in terms of active treatment. One of the most valuable things you can give her is your time. Listen to her explanation of symptoms and worries, and her story/experience as a patient.

Patient issues

- You need to allow this patient time to express her ideas, concerns and expectations about her diagnosis and its perceived implications.

- The psychological impact of having nursed her sister with the same disease, and no doubt patients at the nursing home with terminal problems, will probably have left her with a lot of preconceived ideas and worries:
  – is there any depression or anxiety because of the disease, the pain or other issues?
  – does she think that pain equals progression of the cancer?

- What support is there?
  – is she trying to protect those close to her and ending up bottling up everything that is worrying her, so that she is left feeling isolated?

- Has she thought about death (more than likely)?
  – the pain may mean that this has been on her mind more than ever, possibly fearing the event
  – what sort of death did her sister have?
  – it may be that fear is increasing the perception of the pain.

- Social and financial issues:
  – does she have financial worries or support?
  – if she still has a mortgage, can this be paid off?
  – are friends reluctant to visit or visiting too much?

- Spiritual feelings:
  – often beliefs become more significant as death approaches
  – does she need any help to contact the appropriate minister?

- Legal issues:
  – is she prepared? Has she thought about preparing an advance statement or directive?
  – has she made a will? And is she aware of things like inheritance tax?

Doctor issues

- Pain — on the face of it this is the main issue, and it needs to be fully explored as appropriate:
  - 80% of cancer patients have more than one type of pain
  - 30% have more than three types.

- History and examination:
  - ?ascites (needs tapping)
  - ?jaundice (liver capsule pain)
  - ?tumour bulk
  - ?bony metastases
  - ?subacute bowel obstruction.

Presumably suitability for chemotherapy, radiotherapy and surgery was assessed and discussed at the time of diagnosis. Sometimes it is worth reconsidering the options.

- Conventional treatment:
  - increased analgesia (oral, patch, subcutaneous, etc.)
  - anti-emetics or laxatives may be necessary
  - antidepressants, steroids, dietary supplements, etc.

- Complementary treatment:
  - acupuncture (for pain and nausea)
  - relaxation therapy
  - homeopathy, etc.

- The Gold Standards Framework (Last days of life/care of the dying pathway):
  - this pathway is being increasingly integrated, and is used to support patients and their families in the last few days of life. If it has not already done so, is this an area the practice could target?

- Legal issues:
  - have the issues of resuscitation, or advance directive been discussed?

- Confidentiality:
  - although there may be family around, the patient may not want to involve them — be aware of this.

- Accessibility:
  - who will provide palliative care out of hours? Will it be you, your local co-operative, or maybe the hospice?
  - communication is essential if care is to be handed over
  - is there a practice policy on palliative care — does there need to be one?
  - accessibility to other services in the primary healthcare team is also important.

- Bereavement counselling:
  - for both Margaret and her family.

- Cultural and ethical issues surrounding her care:
  - what treatment does she and doesn't she want (autonomy, non-maleficence)?
  - how does she want to die? Are there any special requests for how her body is treated, etc.?
- Personal implications:
  - you have to deal with your own grief
  - such cases can take up a lot of time, which can be either fulfilling/rewarding or irritating
  - housekeeping is very important (e.g. talking to partners).

Primary healthcare team issues

- Macmillan nurse involvement (if it has not already been arranged, now might be a good time for a referral).
- District nurse (e.g. for support, syringe drivers, enemas, etc.).
- Physiotherapy (for maintaining mobility, loan of TENS machine, acupuncture, etc.).
- Community psychiatric nurse (if considered helpful in the situation can be a useful resource).
- Social services:
  - DS1500 and benefits
  - home aids (also occupational therapy).

Written question 7

A woman attends for a pill check. As you are taking her blood pressure you notice various bruises up her arm. How would you tackle such a finding?

This is a question on domestic violence. Although in this case you are witness to what seems to be the physical manifestation of abuse, always be aware of the emotional and mental aspects, too.

Up to 25% of women (and one in six men) will experience domestic violence at some point in their life. It is a problem that is under-identified in the UK for a multitude of reasons.

Patient issues

- Is this her (not so) hidden agenda? (She would have known about the bruises and that you would have to take her blood pressure.) Is she looking for help?
- Does she have low self-esteem, depression, anxiety, etc.?
- Are you her last resort? What has she tried up until now?
- Are there children involved? Are they at risk? Do social services, health visitors or child protection teams need to be informed and involved?

- What other fears does she have?
  - social isolation
  - financial
  - her own anger and ability to exact revenge
  - the risk of permanent injury
  - the safety and wellbeing of her children
  - the shame of people finding out, etc.

Doctor issues

A good place to start is to ask
BMJ 2002; 324: 271–4

This paper found that most women welcome inquiries, but that doctors and nurses rarely ask. They also found that there was a strong association with anxiety and depression.

General practitioner management of intimate partner abuse and the whole family: qualitative study
BMJ 2004; 328: 618–21

This was a triangulated qualitative study comparing 28 GPs (on a study day) and their reported management with the current recommendations. The conclusion was that guidelines for managing whole families should be developed, children's welfare should always be considered, separate partner referral to services should be considered and GPs should seek help from specialist family violence agencies.

- Make a thorough assessment of the patient:
  - physical and psychological factors, alcohol and drug use
  - social history, support and current situation.

- Confidentiality – this is an important point to emphasise. If your patient doesn't want any input, unless a child's welfare is at stake, you cannot force it on her.

- Notes:
  - you need excellent documentation of injuries witnessed, history of events (if forthcoming) and your assessment, in case of future court cases against the partner
  - consider medical illustration for photographic evidence.

- Learning needs:
  - is this an area you need to brush up on?
  - it raises issues such as communication skills, ethics (of the decisions you are about to make), human rights
  - are you aware of the local services available to be able to advise the patient?

- Accessibility:
  - this woman needs a point of contact (e.g. the police, Women's Aid National Helpline, etc.) if she runs into further problems.

- Is the abusing partner a patient?
  - are there psychological, anger, alcohol problems that you could help with to improve the situation?

Practice issues

- Is there need for a practice protocol and update on domestic violence?

- Is there written information available for patients?

  - this is mainly about helplines (be aware of the implications if this is found at home)
  - should this be on a notice board/in the toilets (male as well as female)?

- Screening is an issue repeatedly raised. We know that patients who are affected want to be asked, and those who are not affected don't mind being asked. Tact and diplomacy are helpful attributes. The issue of screening raises numerous points, for example:
  - time (another thing to screen for in a 10-minute consultation)
  - selective screening (on clinical suspicion)
  - training (in communication skills)
  - the abuse may involve rape and meticulous collection of samples (involvement of a police surgeon would be needed).

Could health professionals screen women for domestic violence?
Systematic review
BMJ **2002; 324: 314–18**

This review found that 50–75% of women felt that screening was acceptable, but only 30% of family doctors (mostly in American studies) felt that it was acceptable. Only two studies showed a decrease in physical and non-physical abuse with intervention. It concluded that it would be premature to introduce screening at this stage.

Primary healthcare team issues

- Role of community psychiatric nurse or family counselling services.

- Health visitor and social services may be aware, or may need to be informed (especially with regard to child welfare).

Written question 8

A young Chinese student has recently registered with your practice, having come to the UK with her husband to study. She comes to you requesting some more of the herbal medicine that she was given for pelvic pain and 'narrowed tubes'. How would you deal with this situation?

The boundaries between alternative and Western conventional medicine are becoming less defined. It is just as important to understand herbal medicines and their side effects as it is for any other drug. Unfortunately, reliable literature on some treatments is hard to come by.

Patient issues

You need to explore this woman's history further.

- What was previously investigated and what did she understand (e.g. pelvic inflammatory disease, sexually transmitted diseases, infertility, etc.)?
- What exactly is she taking and for what purpose?
- Are she and her husband trying to conceive? If so, is the remedy teratogenic and should she stop using it altogether? It is important to counsel her appropriately.
- How is she funding her study?
- Are there financial problems? Is that why she has turned to you for a script rather than obtaining it from a Chinese herbalist?
- Is there a second reason for coming to the UK? Is there a hidden medical agenda (e.g. the need for infertility treatment)?

Doctor issues

- Is it possible to access medical records (with the patient's consent)?
- Is it necessary to repeat certain tests (e.g. swabs, ultrasound scans, laparoscopy and dye, etc.)?
- Is there a need to engage an interpreter to understand her history correctly?
- If you are not familiar with the treatment and there are no medical issues you need to address, is there a reputable Chinese herbalist in the area that you can recommend to her? This would depend on the patient's wish for treatment and her ability to afford it.

Cultural ideals

Be aware of the cultural differences, particularly in terms of health, diagnosis and treatments. Not all countries are as strict as the UK about requiring documentation before you can set up in practice, and this has a knock-on effect on what patients come to expect.

Ethical principles

Treating patients who are taking other medications can lead to problems. Although the patient's autonomy is to be respected, if you are not familiar with treatment, how can you be sure you are not doing your patient harm or neglecting further necessary investigation?

Written question 9

You receive a discharge letter about the death of Fred, an elderly patient, from a haemorrhagic stroke. Fred had been on warfarin for atrial fibrillation, which you had diagnosed and started treatment for 3 years previously. What implications does this death have?

Atrial fibrillation increases the risk of stroke. Several trials have shown that anticoagulation in this group can decrease the risk of stroke by up to 70%, but there are risks and management implications of anticoagulation therapy. Not only that, there has been at least one meta-analysis that advocates the use of aspirin over warfarin (in non-rheumatic atrial fibrillation) in terms of outcome and iatrogenic complications.

The patient's family

- Find out whether they would like (from yourself or another doctor at the practice):
  - a bereavement visit
  - an explanation of the treatment Fred was on (discussed openly, not in a defensive manner), and why a potentially harmful treatment was started.

- Listen to their worries/concerns:
  - about the stroke, treatment and circumstances of death
  - about their grief
  - about any potential issues; try to pre-empt any complaint.

Doctor issues

- Review the individual case:
  - was treatment appropriate and considered in full by the doctor and patient? Was this documented?
  - was the warfarin well monitored and controlled?
  - had there been any prescribing issues that may have potentiated the effects of the warfarin?
  - was Fred of sound mind (i.e. taking his tablets appropriately and not likely to overdose)?
  - were there any other untreated risk factors (e.g. hypertension, mitral stenosis, etc.)?

- If there are any discrepancies, are they worthy of a significant event analysis?

- You may need to acknowledge your own sense of guilt and responsibility, especially if you had gone out of your way to convince the patient that warfarin was a good thing to prevent a stroke.

- Personal ethics of such a situation (i.e. non-maleficence):
  - ethics are always interesting to explore. Although the patient was treated and advised for the correct reasons, the outcome is not as one would want.

Practice issues

- Is there a policy (if not, does there need to be one?) for the following:
  - when to consider warfarin?
  - monitoring warfarin (a register and who doses the patient)?
  - auditing compliance?
  - auditing outcome (e.g. mortality)?
- Complaint procedure:
  - although treatment was (presumably) justified, it would be an appropriate time to update the complaints procedure and educate staff appropriately.

Primary healthcare team issues

- Consider their roles in the following:
  - bereavement within the family (e.g. community psychiatric nurse, district nurse, health visitor)
  - monitoring bloods (district nurse/phlebotomist)
  - elderly health checks (i.e. dementia issues); as a doctor doing a drug review/ consultation, we are easily fooled into believing that a patient has their wits about them when it could be a completely different story at home
  - primary care trust – mandatory reporting of deaths of patients on warfarin.

Written question 10

One of your receptionists comes through red-faced to tell you that a patient of the practice is being verbally aggressive and threatening physical violence if she is not seen by a doctor immediately. There are no notes on the patient as she has only joined the practice recently, having moved into the area. What issues does this raise?

This is quite obviously a question about safety, violence and aggression. Violence in general practice has been on the increase. There are various theories on why this is so, including modern-day life stresses, increased patient expectations, alcohol and drugs.

A Medical Defence Union survey found that two-thirds of doctors feared that they might be physically assaulted at work. Out of 1,044 respondents, 23% had been physically assaulted in the previous 5 years.

This has prompted a Government 'NHS zero tolerance campaign', which was launched in October 1999. It set a target to reduce the incidence of violence by 20% by 2001 and by 30% by 2003 (as yet there are no figures to indicate success). Despite this, GPs are failing to report violent incidents as they feel that nothing would be done about it.

Primare care trusts should offer a safe place for doctors to see violent patients. In some areas, co-operatives are employing doctors to provide this service.

Patient issues

- Why does she need to see a doctor so urgently?
- Why has she moved to the area?

- Are there psychological or dependence issues (alcohol or drugs)?

- Does she have children? If so, is her violence an indication that they could be at risk?

- Is this a typical pattern of behaviour for this patient?

- Is this patient aware of your policy on violence and aggression? (It is possible that this is a way of expressing frustration and she in fact has learning difficulties, i.e. cannot read – not that this should be used to excuse the behaviour.)

Practice issues

As employers, we are responsible for ensuring that our staff are safe at work. The Health and Safety Act 1974 highlights the need for risk assessment and training.

- Layout of the room (involvement of the police with security issues):
  - door opening outwards
  - positioning and type of furniture
  - sharps, needles, equipment, etc., kept out of sight
  - panic buttons easily accessible.

- Protocols:
  - on safety issues and zero tolerance
  - training (signs to look for, methods to use to dissipate tension)
  - involvement of other members of staff (e.g. chaperone)
  - involve the primary healthcare team and primary care trust, and possibly the police.

- Security:
  - consider CCTV
  - consider personal alarms
  - consider panic buttons
  - avoid unnecessary danger (e.g. having only one member of staff on duty).

- Significant event analysis:
  - is it worthwhile using this particular case?
  - involve all, using the session for education and debriefing.

- Training:
  - communication – could such a situation have been avoided with non-aggressive conflict resolution?
  - break-away techniques
  - signs of pending violence.

- Review the appointment system:
  - is this at fault? Are too few appointments causing frustration for staff as well as patients?

- Environment:
  - try to have a comfortable waiting area (not just a call screen to look at).

- Information:
  - keep patients informed of delays
  - share information on dangerous patients among staff. If patients are violent or aggressive, they forego some of their rights to confidentiality in the name of safety for your staff.

Doctor issues

- Safety for you, your staff and other patients is paramount. Do the police need to be called in this situation?
- Most people will settle down if they get to see a doctor, but:
  - is it safe to see this person alone?
  - do you need a chaperone?
- Be aware of safety issues:
  - remove potential missiles or problems (e.g. tie, stethoscope, sharps, etc.)
  - install panic buttons
  - again, room layout. Try to make sure the patient is not between you and the door.
- You need to make a medical and psychiatric assessment:
  - what is the problem (unlikely to be a true emergency)?
  - is it a workable problem?
- You will need excellent negotiating and communication skills, especially if she is requesting something you are not prepared to do:
  - is this a learning need?
- You need to document the incident and the consultation well and consider tagging the computer records.
- Do you feel it necessary to remove the patient, in the name of zero tolerance? This would have implications for:
  - other practices in the area
  - her attitude towards doctors in the future, etc.

  If you do decide to remove the patient from your list you need to contact the police before the primary care trust in order to obtain an incident number. If you don't, the 7-day rule will apply and the patient will be entitled to medical services within that time.
- You have a duty of care medically and ethically to this patient, but not at the expense of safety.

Miscellaneous issues

- Be aware of the effect such an incident may have on your other patients. It may be unsettling, but could also reinforce the notion that if you are aggressive you will jump to the top of the queue.
- Be aware of the Criminal Injuries Compensation Authority and the NHS Benefit Scheme.

Written question 11

A 35-year-old heterosexual female patient attends with her sister, asking to be referred for donor insemination. She is currently single and seems to be extremely well informed. Under what framework would you approach this question?

You do not have to be an expert in fertility treatment to gain marks in this type of question. This type of consultation wouldn't necessarily fit your typical approach, such is the beauty of general practice!

The main issues to consider would be:

- a medical assessment

- a psychological assessment

- pre-conception counselling

- the welfare of a future child

- legal understanding.

Medical assessment

This would include the following.

- A gynaecological history in relation to expected fertility:
  - period cycle
  - history of sexually transmitted infections
  - previous pregnancies and outcome
  - previous blood tests (e.g. for rubella immunity, HIV, syphilis, etc.)
  - is it worth considering checking ovulation bloods (for example) prior to referral?

- A knowledge of medical and family history:
  - are there any medications that need to be altered because of teratogenicity, or illnesses that may affect outcome (in terms of carrying a foetus to term)?
  - does the patient smoke or drink alcohol to excess?
  - are there any family medical problems (e.g. diabetes, gene disorders) that may impact on either the pregnancy or the child?
  - are the family aware of your patient's plans?

Psychological assessment

This would need to consider the following areas.

- Why is your patient wanting to take such drastic action rather than choosing the father of her child, i.e. in a consenting relationship?

- Why is there such a need for a child at this point – is she emotionally stable to cope with the life changes?

- Are there personal attachment issues that may not explain the request but have potentially damaging effects for a future child?
- Has your patient considered the chance of future relationships and natural conception, and how that would impact on her current choice?

Pre-conception counselling

This would include the following.

- Smoking, alcohol, lifestyle and folic acid advice.
- Consideration of immunity screening (e.g. rubella) prior to conception.
- Consideration of the above factors that may impact on a pregnancy.

Understanding the welfare of a future child

This is very difficult, given the snapshot we have of a person's life when they are with us, and the attitudes people can convey that may be completely contrary to who they are and how they live their life.

Legally, a fertility unit is prohibited from offering treatment if there would be a justified concern for the protection of that child. There is also an issue around future relationships and how they might impact on the single-parent unit.

Legal understanding

The Human Fertilisation and Embryology Authority (HFEA) is a statutory non-departmental public body that grants licences for the following assisted-conception techniques:

- *in-vitro* fertilisation
- intracytoplasmic sperm injection
- preimplantation genetic diagnosis
- sperm donation
- egg donation
- embryo donation
- surrogacy.

In this case, the sperm would be donated, and if the woman went on to have a successful pregnancy, the child would need to be registered with the HFEA.

The HFEA is also responsible for issuing guidance on consent, counselling and welfare of the child.

The HFEA Act (1990) requires that a person must have 'a suitable opportunity to receive proper counselling on the implications of taking on the proposed steps'.

Whatever your own moral ethics or religious beliefs in such a situation, you would be unwise to refuse to refer this patient (privately, as this would not be available on the NHS). Although it would be the responsibility of the gynaecologist to whom this woman is referred, if you are able, it would be helpful to discuss the steps that you expect to happen, and the treatment options.

Written question 12

> You have been allocated a number of asylum seekers. A woman comes to see you in surgery with her son (who is translating) and her daughter (who appears to have learning disabilities). She is requesting hormone replacement therapy (HRT). How do you approach the consultation?

Consultations involving language barriers and cultural issues are common in primary (and secondary) care. There are several issues raised here and they cannot all be dealt with in one consultation.

Many asylum seekers will have telephone numbers for people who will translate for them over the telephone. This can be very useful, but brings into question the issue of confidentiality and real understanding. You generally will have no knowledge of the person who is translating.

Patient issues

- Why HRT?
  - Was the woman using HRT previously? If not, what has she read and why is she requesting it now?
- Menopause.
  - Is she menopausal or does she have symptoms that suggest she is perimenopausal? If this is the case, is it appropriate for her age?
  - What are her periods like?
  - Are there any risk factors for osteoporosis?
  - Does she need contraception?
  - Can she fully understand the risks vs. the benefits given the method of translating?
- Other issues.
  - The psychological impact of status, a new country with higher costs of living, different cultures, etc.
  - Other medical/health promotion issues (e.g. chronic diseases and screening (cervical cytology), vaccinations, etc.).

Cultural issues

The fact that her son is translating for her, especially when talking about gynaecological issues, may not be appropriate. Thus the information you think you are getting across and receiving in return may not be accurate.

Further family/social factors

- Are the children now in school (given that they are new to the area)? Are they coping, given the perceived challenges and the different culture? It is sometimes helpful to ascertain why asylum is being sought.

- Has her daughter had an educational needs assessment or is she already on a Statement, given the impression you have (i.e. that of a learning disability)? Are there related medical issues that would need addressing?

- Is there any other adult support (e.g. father, family)?

- Is there an income?

- Understanding the circumstances behind a person seeking asylum leads to a better understanding, which may in turn improve their care. Certain problems, especially the psychological impact, can be pre-empted (to some extent) and addressed.

Doctor issues

- You need to be happy that the information you are receiving and trying to relay is accurate.

- Confidentiality – are you happy that translation by her son is improving the care and understanding for this patient and not putting her at a disadvantage?

- Does she need contraceptive services or to be entered into the cervical screening programme?

- You have a duty of care to the children. New patients will need new patient checks to ensure all their needs are met to the best of your ability with the given resources.

Practice issues

- Is there an HRT protocol and leaflet? If not, is this an area to develop?

- Is there a new demand that would warrant translation of information/leaflets into another language (e.g. for cervical screening there are versions in many different languages available on the Department of Health's website)?

- Is there someone in the primary care trust who would be able to translate?

- What is the social service network like for those people who need further, ongoing help?

The MRCGP oral examination

This may well be the most nerve-wracking part of the exam. There is no anonymity as with the written paper, nor is editing allowed as with the video. This is you, warts and all.

The oral takes place a few weeks after the written paper. For my colleagues and I this worked well, as we found it was necessary to adopt a completely different approach. With our (made-up) questions we fired them blindly at each other only to find we had to be quick thinking and professional, and that wisecracks didn't really work! We didn't think it was going too badly until we watched the RCGP video. Despite all our time in medicine we knew almost nothing about management, teambuilding, what qualities make a good chairperson, etc. We certainly didn't know the lingo to make ourselves sound convincing!

The oral exam is designed to determine how you will perform in real life (it is incredibly good practice for future interviews). It tests your communication skills, decision making and professional values in four main areas:

- care of patients
- working with colleagues
- the social role of general practice
- the doctor's personal responsibilities.

The exam consists of two consecutive 20-minute orals, each conducted by two examiners. There is a 5-minute break between the two parts, giving the examiners time to mark your performance. Each 20-minute exam will consist of approximately five questions.

Most of the time the examiners are pleasant and will try to help you if you are struggling, or push you if you are doing well. Some people have reported a 'good cop, bad cop' style, try not to be fazed if this happens.

One final tip: remember to dress smartly and polish your shoes!

I have put together 10 questions, again with my thoughts on how you might approach the answers. I have used a number of management and team building books as well as information from local courses (Pioneer 2005). Try to practise in pairs and make it like the exam. If an obvious question is raised from the answer, ask it, and if something is not clear, ask the person to explain it (that goes for the person asking the question as well as the one answering it). It is worth noting that the White Paper on care outside hospitals is due to be published (this will contain proposals and statements of Government policy) and will become topical in the oral exam. You don't have to talk willy-nilly for 5 minutes on each question. If you reach a natural pause, that's fine – the examiner will ask you something else.

Oral question I

A patient you have been treating is now in the end stages of heart failure. He cannot even wash himself without becoming extremely short of breath. If he were to ask you to help him end things quickly and peacefully, how would you respond?

This is obviously a question on euthanasia, which is still a crime in the UK. The GMC has recently issued a statement in support of there being no change in the law, especially in light of the advances in palliative care.

There are a number of issues that could be discussed.

Quality of life

Presumably for this patient it is poor. It is important to find out what is the worst thing for him (e.g. lack of dignity, feeling unwell, being a burden, etc.).

- Listen, and empathise (if appropriate), to what his issues and health beliefs are.

- Anything you offer him should be aimed at improving the quality of life he has left.

Empathy is described in Gillies' Occasional Paper as 'a complex multi-dimensional concept that has moral, cognitive, emotive and behavioural components'. Morse described four components of empathy:

1 Emotive – the ability to subjectively experience/share another's psychological state.

2 Moral – an internal altruistic force that motivates the practice of empathy.

3 Cognitive – the helper's intellectual ability to understand a person's perspective from a distance.

4 Behavioural – communicative response to convey understanding.

Medical treatment options

These are aimed at maximising heart failure treatment. Any unnecessary treatment should be stopped.

- Diuretics – for example, could his renal function tolerate metolazone or spironolactone?

- Nitrates/ACE inhibitors.

- Beta-blockers are unlikely to be warranted at this stage but are worth considering.

- Home oxygen – for symptomatic relief.

- Morphine, diazepam, etc., in small doses are often very helpful.

- Is he becoming clinically depressed and does this need treatment?

- Does he need an acute admission?

Primary healthcare team issues

- Occupational therapists, district nurses and social services should all be involved, with the patient's consent. The counsellor may also be of benefit. Most services will now work with the care of the dying pathway in such circumstances, despite it being developed for cancer patients.

- In some areas, if there are beds available, a hospice may take such patients for respite or palliation.

- Teamwork and good communication are fundamental to successful care, especially the hand-over to the out-of-hours team. Remember that the most important member of the team is the patient.

Euthanasia

As much as you may empathise with your patient, euthanasia would be viewed in a legal context as murder. Patients usually understand this and don't pressure their doctors further.

Advanced directives

Is it an appropriate time to discuss eventualities (e.g. in the event of a cardiac arrest). To arrange an advanced directive, the patient would need legal council and have to be fully informed of all possible eventualities. In such cases, it is important to encourage the patient to discuss the directives with their family.

Cultural issues

- What religion is your patient? Would he appreciate input from the local church, mosque, etc.?
- Is part of the reason he is requesting euthanasia because of personal/cultural beliefs about cleanliness and nursing?

The examiners, if you have not already answered, may push you on whether or not you would help this man to die. Given the legal implications, whatever your view, it would be prudent to answer 'no', possibly adding that you would help to keep him as comfortable as possible with the appropriate support.

This question could easily apply to patients with cancer, multiple sclerosis, motor neurone disease, etc. As death is certain for us all, this will remain topical for some time yet.

It is important to show that you empathise with the patient and will do your best to maximise the quality of time he has left, but that you also understand the legal boundaries.

Oral question 2

What do you understand by the term 'medical ethics'?

Ethical reasoning is a branch of philosophy that deals with right and wrong. In the UK, law is either statute (acts passed by Parliament) or common (law formed on precedent and judicial interpretation of statute).

GPs need to be aware of both legal and ethical frameworks on medical issues and decision making.

Discussions are currently being formed into two theoretical approaches.

1 *Deontological theories* — the view that correct actions should be based on our duties, and that whether the action is right or wrong is determined by the action itself rather than the consequences.

2 *Consequentialism* — the view that the right action in a situation should be based on the value of the results or consequence of that action.

Getting it right in the consultation: Hippocrates' problem; Aristotle's answer (Occasional Paper 86, John Gillies) was published in August 2005 and will probably become part of your examiner's own reading (it is a paper that will help you understand some of the philosophical discussions).

The four model principle

This allows analysis of a problem, but not necessarily its resolution.

1 *Beneficence* — the principle that doctors should only do good for their patients.

2 *Non-maleficence* — the principle that a doctor should do no harm.

3 *Justice* — the principle that scarce healthcare resources should be shared fairly. This is distributive rather than criminal justice.

4 *Autonomy* — the principle that all patients should have self-determination over their own decisions. A fully autonomous decision should be informed, competent and not coerced.

The four moral theory

1 *Theory of virtue* — describes innate character attributes that are either good or bad.

2 *Theory of duties* — rationally based rules of moral conduct. In the UK, these rules are set out as GMC regulations.

3 *Theory of utility* — describes what is morally good in terms of 'greatest good for the greatest number'.

4 *Theory of rights* — describes social relationships between people such that some have an obligation to provide a service to others based on intrinsic right.

If you cite one ethical model and show that you understand it, you will have done well. The obvious follow-on question is 'Do you know any other ethical models?' If you don't, say that you don't know them well enough to explain them. You've found a model that works for you, and that is generally what you try to apply to help you to analyse a situation (or something along those lines!). If you can remember other models then certainly discuss them, but try to do it in context.

Oral question 3

Do you think prescribing rationale has changed over the past 40 years?

- All the evidence suggests that the answer to the question is yes.
- The availability of drugs has increased (different drug classes as well as drugs with the same class effect).
- We have an ageing society with the associated diseases and problems. This will often mean multiple drug regimens to reduce morbidity, mortality and improve quality of life. The average elderly person now has 8.8 items on repeat prescription.
- We as doctors are more aware of evidence-based prescribing issues, as well as the fact that there is more research on the safety profile of a given drug.
- Much of our work is now about primary prevention (e.g. coronary heart disease risk and the use of statins).
- There has been a rise in different types of advertising of drugs available on prescription and over the counter. This increases patient awareness (a good thing), but it also increases the financial burden on the NHS (a bad thing, especially when a patient is requesting a drug that is unproven).
- Even in the absence of advertising, patient awareness and demand are increasing as information becomes increasingly accessible on the Internet.
- GPs are now prescribing and monitoring drugs that were previously only available in secondary care (e.g. fertility drugs). This obviously impacts on a GP's drug budget and there are medicolegal pitfalls about prescribing specialist drugs.
- Our knowledge of antibiotic resistance is increasing, and GPs have altered prescribing habits accordingly. Another example of changing prescribing habits would be for blood pressure control.
- External factors that impact on GP prescribing include the following:
  - personal experience (adverse outcomes and successes)
  - National Service Frameworks and NICE
  - local primary care trust guidance
  - local consultant preferences as patients are discharged on certain drugs
  - patient pressure
  - pharmacological companies (representatives, drug deals for dispensing practices)
  - local educational meetings and guest speakers.

This question would lead nicely on to questions such as the following.

- Do you think nurse/pharmacist prescribing will impact on GP prescribing budgets/ PACT data?
- Do you think nurse prescribing will undo the hard work of public health and GPs in encouraging self-management of minor ailments and the reductions achieved in antibiotic prescribing?
- How would you go about implementing nurse prescribing in your practice?

All of the above questions raise issues such as:

- whether nurses want to expand their role (the first question to answer)
- training issues for supplementary/independent prescribing
- the drawing up of protocols and patient group directives
- supervision and accessibility of GPs
- audit
- the issue of nurse practitioners having their own lists, especially in inner-city areas where there is often difficulty recruiting GPs.

The Royal College of General Practitioners is in favour of nurse prescribing by nurses who wish to develop these skills, but recognises the need for training and support. There must be safeguards for nurses with revalidation.

The CROWN Review (1999) recommended the following for extended nurse prescribing:

- a period of supervised practice
- drugs to which 'new prescribers' have access would be subject to expert clinical pharmacology and safety vetting
- the need for training and education.

Oral question 4

How do you think flexible training and employment will affect general practice?

This does not have to apply to doctors only, but can also include nursing, reception and office staff, depending on how you want to frame your answer.

Currently, more than 50% of a medical school intake is female. Women represent over 30% of the GP workforce, and the numbers appear to be increasing. Although not solely a female issue (other than the need for maternity leave!), family life and childcare impact greatly on the need for work to be flexible in order to get the most from employees.

Advantages of flexible training and employment

- It allows flexible career choices.
- It makes a profession more appealing because of that flexibility.
- It improves personal fulfilment (e.g. the decision of quality versus income).
- GPs and medically trained professionals may be encouraged to stay in the profession (i.e. work can fit in with family life).
- Cynically, it means that the NHS gets more for its money, as part-time workers will virtually always work more than the hours for which they are paid (as do

people who work full time, but there are more hours on to which the work can encroach for part-time staff).

- It can improve time management and organisation, as it is less easy to put things off until tomorrow.

- It will hopefully reduce stress, burnout and the number of people who retire early.

- It may reduce the amount of sick leave taken.

- It may reduce the number of people who would have to retrain because they had taken time out to raise a family.

- It would increase the number of people employed and so decrease unemployment and benefits claimed (thinking in terms of office and reception staff).

Disadvantages of flexible training and employment

- If people work part time, there will need to be even more doctors and staff.

- The overall cost for the NHS will increase (training, pay, national insurance, superannuation, sick pay, maternity pay, etc.).

- Access for the patients may become an issue, especially if a practice works on the principle that doctors see their own registered patients. This would obviously disadvantage the patients of the doctor working part time.

- There may be less job satisfaction, for example if you are caring for a palliative care patient and they need care when you are not available, this may affect continuity and treatment success.

- There may be practice issues (hence the value of a well-considered practice agreement detailing even the smallest points on the distribution of workload) where a full-time partner feels that a part-time partner ought to put in more time, or is even jealous that they cannot go part time.

- You may not be at work when certain meetings take place. This raises the need for agendas and good minute keeping and circulation.

Oral question 5

Do you think disease registers have a place in modern-day healthcare?

The answer to this question is yes, particularly for chronic disease management (they are also part of the new GMS contract for certain diseases). However, disease registers raise numerous issues for patients, doctors, nurses and administration staff.

Advantages of disease registers

- Disease registers help to target patient groups, e.g. diabetics, asthmatics, coronary heart disease, etc., to ensure they are receiving the best care.

- It is easier to:
  - audit management success against set criteria
  - recall patients for follow-up
  - communicate with secondary care and the primary care trust.

- It may mean patients get better care (although this is not a foregone conclusion):
  - guidelines are developed (or adopted) in keeping with evidence
  - clinics are able to focus on specific problems (so disease areas are not just glossed over when consulting for a sore throat).

- Although initially the process of setting up a new register can be time-consuming, once complete it should be relatively simple to keep accurate and to update.

Disadvantages of disease registers

- Doctors and nurses may become so preoccupied with ticking boxes that they forget the patient and lose some of their own clinical application skills.

- Templates and keeping the register up to date can be time-consuming if they are not simple.

- Disease registers do not assess quality of care.

- There are consent and confidentiality issues for the patients (by virtue of their being on a register).

- It is necessary to ensure that all doctors and nurses are completing relevant areas (i.e. that there is continued motivation).

- If a practice is not computerised/computer literate, this is an arduous task. Although part of the NHS plan is that all practices be computerised, this does not necessarily mean that all practices will make good use of those systems.

- If you have patients who are non-compliant and disinterested (e.g. in their HbA_{1C} levels), and have not reached the point where they wish to be 'educated', then they may affect your figures, which may in turn affect your pay. There needs to be some way to take compliance into account, depending on what you want to achieve with your register (e.g. exclusion reporting in specific instances).

Oral question 6

What do you understand by quality within the NHS?

Quality is all about standards (of all things, not just clinical care), and being able to give people (patients and staff) what they need as well as what they want. It does this at the lowest possible cost (i.e. is economical).

A good framework for standards is the GMC's *Good Medical Practice*. Although revalidation should be part of the overall equation in achieving quality of care, it is only a small part of it.

Quality includes the following:

- development:
  - of staff and the organisation in pre-defined areas
  - of new methods

- objective measurements:
  - audit
  - quarterly statistics
  - satisfaction questionnaires, etc.

- productivity:
  - improved satisfaction that is economical.

Or, alternatively:

- patient quality:
  - what do they want from the services?

- professional quality:
  - education and training issues
  - revalidation

- management quality:
  - helps to ensure efficient, productive use of resources available.

Clinical governance should feature somewhere in your discussion about controlling quality.

This question could lead on to the following question: 'Why is quality important?'

- It improves satisfaction all around (patients/clients and staff).

- Work is more enjoyable and less frustrating.

- It increases productivity and control.

- It reduces unnecessary costs, and this increases potential income.

- It reduces the likelihood of complaints and negligence claims.

- It improves staff morale and interprofessional co-operation.

- It makes recruitment and retention easier in a competitive labour market.

- It avoids duplication (e.g. of administrative tasks).

- It enhances reputation, which is good for morale and business in a competitive market.

- It creates a focus for development strategies – a service cannot be 'all things to all people', so it is important to single out groups of people for a particular service.

Issues to look at when determining quality features

- Competence:
  - of employees
  - appropriate skills and training to perform as you would expect.

- Communication:
  - with clients
  - not just in a consultation context, but also ways to keep them informed of changes and listen to their concerns (e.g. notice boards, newsletters, a website).

- Credibility:
  - honesty towards staff and patients (probity).

- Security:
  - physical safety, confidentiality, etc.

- Courtesy:
  - client orientation of staff
  - polite and friendly staff with the ability to listen.

- Access:
  - a service needs to be readily accessible.

- Reliability:
  - this ties in with credibility.

- Physical tangibles:
  - the environment and appearance of the staff reflect the people who work there and their employers.

Oral question 7

As a GP, how would you facilitate good methods of communication between staff?

Effective communication is essential for a team to be successful. It saves time and reduces unnecessary frustrations.

There are many different methods of communication:

- verbal

- message books/notes

- computer (email and message screens)

- meetings, with minutes that are accessible, distributed or displayed

- appraisals

- a complaints procedure.

Ultimately, effective communication will result in effective teamwork, and better productivity and morale.

Whatever method is used for a particular issue needs to be reliable, and will work better if it is a method that is agreed by all users (i.e. there is some ownership).

Part of making communication effective is creating a dynamic team. This involves leadership skills and getting to know people.

There are three key factors common to all effective teams:

1 identification of roles so that there is no confusion

2 having effective and efficient processes in place

3 maintaining a high level of morale.

Building and evolving that team involve the following:

- honesty about current effectiveness

- tackling problems (including personality clashes) head on and working through them

- being prepared to learn new skills as a group.

You mentioned meetings as a method of communication. What do you think distinguishes a good meeting from the not so good?

Meetings need to have a purpose and a conclusion. There needs to be consideration to timing, objectives, venue and the people who should be included. Meetings may need to occur regularly, and there also needs to be an effective chair with good facilitation.

John Cleese's *Meetings, Bloody Meetings* gives a short, sensible guide to successful meetings.

1 Plan ahead – what is the meeting for?

2 Pre-notification – the agenda.

3 Preparation – agenda, order of priority and a guide to the time available.

4 Processing:
   – each discussion needs structure
   – the chairperson must understand the group dynamics to help ensure conflict is creative rather than destructive.

5 Putting it on record:
   – summary of events, decisions made and actions to be taken.

Another frame is 'The Four Ds' from *The PCG Team Builder*.

- Define the problem.

- Define the objective in looking for a solution (consensus/vote/delegate to certain members).

- Decide how to effect a successful solution.

- Determine how you will measure success (evaluate ideas against value/benefit, cost, feasibility and resources available).

Tell me more about the chairperson. What do you understand their role to be?

The chairperson's role is to provide a framework, to maintain the focus and to facilitate – getting the best from all members of the team, as well as getting people to work together as a team.

1 Framework:
  – maintain organisation, time keeping
  – identify when things are drifting/going awry
  – generate options to stop people becoming blinkered
  – set standards (firm but fair).

2 Focus on the issue at hand:
  – clarify points, summarise
  – deal with time wasting.

3 Facilitation:
  – allow flexibility and freedom for expression of views
  – understand others and listen
  – remain unbiased and neutral/impartial
  – encourage co-operation
  – recognise that it is a team effort and that the chairperson cannot make the team effective on their own
  – be sensitive and respectful.

Another summary would be:

- communicate

- control

- co-ordinate

- coax

- compare

- clarify

- concentrate.

Oral question 8

What qualities should a modern GP have?

See the General Medical Council's *Duties of a Doctor* (this is essential reading for the exam and should form part of your answer here). As a profession, we are different from other disciplines. In 1996, McWhinney delivered the Pickles lecture (***Br J Gen Pract* 1996; 46: 433–6**), in which he suggested that the four main differences were as follows.

- We define ourselves in terms of relationships (especially the doctor–patient relationship).

- We think in terms of individual patients.

- We are based on organismic rather than mechanistic metaphors or biology.

- We transcend the dualistic division between body and mind.

Desired qualities

- A modern GP should:
  - be clinically competent
  - be the patient's advocate
  - be a good team player
  - have, or develop, leadership skills
  - be a partner or business person
  - be a reflective practitioner, with self-awareness
  - be open to new ideas, flexible and tolerant
  - be a good teacher
  - be a gatekeeper and resource allocator
  - not be prejudiced
  - avoid discrimination
  - be aware of how their personal beliefs may affect care given/offered
  - treat information with respect and maintain confidentiality
  - be involved in personal and professional growth (revalidation)
  - be able to recognise stresses and hopefully adapt to prevent burnout in themselves, colleagues and employees.

- They should have an ethical and cultural awareness as well as moral principles.

- They may be an employer (or a representative of one) and all this implies (listener, facilitator, fair, enthusiastic, diplomatic).

- They should have an understanding of medicolegal issues.

- They may be involved in research and should always be involved in audit.

- They should be prepared to talk around all of the above issues.

The European Branch of the World Organisation of Family Doctors (WONCA) has developed a new definition of general practice, which is not too dissimilar to the GMC's *Duties of a Doctor*.

Oral question 9

How would you inform a patient that they have bowel cancer following results of investigations you have ordered?

This is a question about good communication skills and the breaking of bad news. The following are the main considerations in such circumstances.

- Have all the facts available, and double-check that they are for the correct person.
- Establish that the patient wants to know more.
- Establish what they already understand.
- Choose the right moment. You will need time, privacy and quiet (i.e. no disturbances).
- Consider whether a relative, partner or friend should be present.
- Keep checking that you are giving the right amount of information and that it is wanted.
- Ask the patient what their main concerns are.
- Find out how they are feeling.
- Don't rush on to treatment. When they are ready, outline a management plan.
- Ensure that there is adequate follow-up and support.
- Throughout, acknowledge and empathise with their feelings, distress, etc.
- Recognise that there will be psychological, social, spiritual and cultural aspects.
- Always try and communicate with the practice team so that everyone is aware of the situation (primary healthcare team meeting, Macmillan involvement, tagging of computer records, etc.).
- Housekeeping (Neighbour's gem).
- Acknowledge your own feelings.

If the patient has little awareness, how would you convey the news without pushing them into denial or provoking overwhelming distress?

- Fire a warning shot, for example 'I'm afraid I have bad news'.
- Try to give them time, so that they ask for the information rather than you forcing the issue.
- Use silence in an active way, not so it becomes uncomfortable, but to allow the patient to process thoughts and questions.

If the patient's relatives ask you not to give the diagnosis to the patient what would you do?

This raises issues of confidentiality. You should ask yourself why you were talking to the relatives rather than the patient in the first place.

There is no right answer here – it depends on the situation.

Be aware that advances in oncology and surgery have meant improved morbidity and mortality in many cancers. Not divulging the information denies the patient these treatments, as well as complicating palliative care with the Macmillan nurses when the time comes.

Oral question 10

How would you go about negotiating a change in working patterns (for example) within your practice?

This could be applied to any number of problems (e.g. rotas, visits, workload). There are various strategies that may encourage people to think about change and take action towards making the change. If people are involved, they are likely to accept and contribute to change. It is important to lead change by example.

The responses that people may have to change are variable:

- some ignore it
- some resist it
- some go along passively
- some plan ahead
- some grasp the opportunity and actively pursue it.

There are five main qualities needed to effect successful change:

- enthusiasm
- energy
- determination
- diplomacy
- foresight.

A simple model for change

1 Where are you now?
   - Motives: financial, psychological, status, reputation, achievement, creativity.
   - Priorities.
   - Talents in relation to change.
   - Time allocation.

2 Where do you want to get to?
   - Define aims, set goals and promote ownership.
   - Agree priorities.
   - Define criteria: success and failure.
   - Define timescale.

3 How are you going to get there?
- Clarify resources.
- Clarify obstructions and helpful factors.
- Conduct a SWOT analysis (strengths, weaknesses, opportunities and threats).
- Select a team and 'create' time for that team.

Domain mapping (Spiegal et al.)

This is quite a useful technique which can encourage all parties with an interest to contribute to an analysis of the effects of any proposed change.

1 Draw six concentric circles.

2 Divide them into as many segments as there are interested parties/stakeholders.

3 Enter details (each detail is applied to each person/segment), such as:
- proposed change
- name of the stakeholder
- current involvement in the situation where change is proposed
- future benefits of the change for each person
- potential costs to each person of proposed change
- potential power of stakeholders to obstruct change.

Good preparation is the key to successful negotiation and change. *MedEconomics* discussed this recently in terms of a 10-point plan.

1 Agree the objectives of your negotiation.

2 Identify the issues for all parties concerned (an issue is something that can be traded).

3 Think about the strengths and weaknesses.

4 Agree the team attitude (this will be defined partly on what role the group is to take after the negotiations).

5 Decide on a strategy.

6 Plan your bargaining position for each issue (if this is feasible, make it known).

7 Prepare your tactics (this is behaviour and actions that bring your attitude to life).

8 Plan your questions and evidence in advance.

9 Agree your alternatives (worst-case scenario planning).

10 Line up your final bargaining models (this could take months; if you have to accept a less-than-ideal position on one issue, trade your concession for a better position on another).

You may be pushed to say how you would make those changes (i.e. implementation) after you have completed the groundwork.

- Involve the relevant people.

- Be thorough in your considerations, and don't just change for the sake of it.

- Make clear, concise plans. As with guidelines, involving the right people creates ownership.

- Have a timescale – be realistic and flexible.

- Have a measure of success/failure (e.g. audit, observation, etc.).

The MRCGP video

The single route (combining the MRCGP and the summative assessment) is by far the most efficient way of doing the consultation skills, but you have to be organised to get it all completed to the correct standard. You *must* familiarise yourself fully with the exam criteria (www.rcgp.org.uk) early in the game. The summative assessment handbook is available from the National Office for Summative Assessment at www.nosa.org.uk (be aware of the changes that will take place by 2007, with the Postgraduate Medical Education and Training Board replacing the JCPTGP).

Seven consultations are required for the MRCGP (these should be the first seven on the tape). Recordings for the summative assessment need to be 2 hours long, with no fewer than eight consultations (you really should do this just in case you fail the MRCGP).

The *MRCGP Video Workbook* contains the following:

- the competencies to be demonstrated (performance criteria)
  - discover the reason for the patient's attendance
  - define the clinical problem(s)
  - explain the problem(s) to the patient
  - address the patient's problem(s)
  - make effective use of the consultation

- detailed instructions for recording consultations

- a video log

- consultation summary forms

- ethical principles.

There is not a great deal of additional direction needed for the video. Working for the rest of the exam will automatically improve your knowledge and performance on tape. You need to start recording early and get used to the process of obtaining signed consent forms (often done in reception so as not to interrupt the flow), taping yourself and critically assessing the consultations. If you are uncomfortable, not only will the patient sense this, but you will also start to make unnecessary mistakes. Using the tapes to identify your learning needs is a good use of your time.

The taping itself is the easy part. You then have to sit down and go through the tapes with the performance criteria to hand. You need to give this your whole attention, as it is the only way to know what points you miss.

Involving your trainer (if you are still a registrar) or colleagues is very important so that you do not become blinkered and less objective. They have a great deal of experience and will help you to identify your unidentified gaps. Discuss how they prefer to view your tapes. Unless you want to demonstrate a specific point it can be a monumental waste of time to go through the ones you already know are unlikely to pass. Your trainer will probably thank you for editing those out and getting straight to the ones you think may be good enough.

It is important to remember to format the tape correctly. At present this needs to be normal speed (short play), the time needs to be visible (clock or screen) and you must have the consent forms to accompany the consultations. Leave yourself plenty of time to edit on to VHS and complete the workbook.

It is worth noting that, depending on your circumstances, you may be able to apply to do the simulated patients instead of the video component. This is one session and, rather like the oral, there is no editing!

Membership by Assessment and Performance (MAP)

This is a relatively new route to gain membership, and has been an option since 1999. It is geared towards GPs who have been in practice for more than 5 years and are able to demonstrate the quality of care they provide. It is expected to be completed over a 2-year period.

You can purchase the MAP handbook from the Royal College of General Practitioners. This sets out the criteria, which are divided into three broad headings: You and Your Practice, Managing Illness, and Learning and Values. There are ten sections to consider:

1 communication and practice

2 accessibility and continuity

3 patient records

4 management of chronic illness

5 management of acute illness

6 prescribing

7 health promotion

8 ethical standards

9 continuing professional development and review of performance

10 consulting skills.

MAP consists of three separate elements:

- a video assessment or simulated surgery
- a portfolio of written evidence (up to nine submissions)
- a practice visit.

Relatively few candidates choose this route, but among those who have passed and written about their experience it seems as though general feelings are similar: it is hard work but the reward is great for practice, patient and doctor.

Exams and courses to consider

While you go through your hospital training you will receive study allowance and grants that can be used to pay for different courses (relevant to general practice, not necessarily the subspecialty you may be doing as part of the rotation at that time).

In your GP registrar year your study leave budget is around £200 (unless your VTS has some extra to use), while in hospital posts it is around £500 (double-check these figures for your trust). You should use the study leave time and money wisely, bearing in mind that if you want to go on revision courses this will use a lot of your registrar allocation, and that certain courses will be free in certain posts (e.g. advanced life support).

Diplomas to consider while going through your hospital posts

DRCOG (Diploma of the Royal College of Obstetricians and Gynaecologists)

This is not essential for general practice, but if you look at job advertisements, you will see that some practices stipulate that they would like applicants to have the diploma. You can only do this exam (MCQs and OSCE) after completing at least 3 months of obstetrics and gynaecology.

If you do want to attempt it, request the information from the college early. If you can time it with your attachment then you will probably find it easier to be motivated, and get significantly more out of the teaching on rounds from your seniors.

> Royal College of Obstetricians and Gynaecologists
> 27 Sussex Place
> London NW1 4RG
> Tel: 020 7772 6200
> www.rcog.org.uk

DFFP (Diploma of the Faculty of Family Planning)

This again is not essential for general practice unless you want to do family planning sessions or fit coils. You can do ad hoc family planning sessions once you have the diploma, while you are still doing either hospital posts or your GP registrar year, which may help you to keep your skills up to date.

Once you have done the DFFP you can do the coil training for the IUD letters of competence (up to five coils in the DFFP training can count towards the 10 that are needed) and the implant training.

If you are considering doing this diploma, you will need to have completed a minimum of 3 months of obstetrics and gynaecology (you can do the theory before this, which is a 3.5-day course if it includes the coil information).

The syllabus and logbook can be viewed on the faculty website (www.ffprhc. org.uk) (under general training committee).

Faculty of Family Planning & Reproductive Health
19 Cornwall Terrace
London NW1 4QP
Tel: 020 7935 7196/7149

DCH (Diploma in Child Health)

This is a detailed diploma involving practical-based sessions as well as the exam. It may be possible to do these sessions while you are in your paediatric job.

Only a few practices seem to be requesting this diploma but, as is often the case, it may be something that tips the balance in your favour when applying for a post.

Royal College of Paediatrics and Child Health
50 Hallam Street
London W1W 6DE
Tel: 020 7307 5600
www.rcpch.ac.uk/

Courses to consider while going through your hospital posts

Advanced life support (ALS)

Ensure that this is up to date before your registrar year and that you have a signed form confirming that you are qualified in ALS. If you are thinking of taking the MRCGP, you have to have proof of basic life support competency, which the ALS training incorporates. Most trusts give this training free of charge for trust employees.

Acupuncture

Many hospital trusts will fund acupuncture courses. Acupuncture is as relevant to general practice as you want to make it. The courses tend to be held at weekends, which means that getting the study leave is not part of the ordeal. A good basic course to ensure you are competent to practise would take about 4 days.

Information can be found in the *British Medical Journal* advertisements. See also:

British Medical Acupuncture Society (BMAS)
Newton House, Newton Lane
Whitley, Warrington WA4 4JA
Tel: 01925 730727
www.medical-acupuncture.co.uk

Some half-day release courses (or within your postgraduate region) will offer the following courses to GP registrars:

- alternative medicine

- ENT

- ophthalmology

- dermatology

- GP management issues

- communication skills.

All of the above, and more, would be time well spent. It is all about developing your own interests and deciding what kind of a service you would like to be able to offer your patients. For example, acupuncture can be done safely in a 10-minute consultation and give incredible relief (a popular misconception is that you need a good half hour).

Courses to consider during your registrar year

Minor surgery

You can pay to go on a minor surgery course while doing your hospital training. GP registrars can usually go on the course without having to pay.

If you want to be signed up by your primary care trust for minor surgery so that you can claim payment for it, then it is necessary to do this course.

The theoretical course is *not* the way in which you will become competent in minor surgery. You will learn this either through your trainer or other colleagues (e.g. dermatologists, surgeons, rheumatologists, etc.) in hospital posts.

Child health surveillance

This is going through a process of change to allow greater involvement of midwives and health visitors in the specific screening at an early age (i.e. neonatal checks, immunisation, etc.).

It is important to check your regional policy as to what is required and whether you have to be on a named list to carry out any surveillance work.

Child health protection (especially the recognition) is an important part of work in primary care and if you have the opportunity to attend one of these courses it would be worthwhile.

Palliative care

Most regions now run palliative care courses, and again GP registrars are not required to pay.

Although palliative care is unlikely to be a huge part of day-to-day life, it will be the one thing that, if you do it well, you will be remembered and respected for.

The course teaches the knowledge base as well as the practical issues (e.g. setting up a syringe driver).

Publications to subscribe to

You should already be receiving the Chief Medical Officer's Updates, the *Drugs and Therapeutics Bulletin*, etc. If you are a member of the British Medical Association you will receive the *British Medical Journal*. Although most information is available online, it can be satisfying to flick through journals and read real paper copies. Your medical library will stock many other journals of interest. The following are currently obtainable free:

Update	www.DoctorUpdate.net
	Tel: 020 8652 8454 (circulation enquiries)
The Practitioner	CMP Information Ltd, Ludgate House,
	Blackfriars Road, London SE1 9UY
	Tel: 0800 626 387
GP (newspaper)	174 Hammersmith Road, London W6 7JP
	www.GPonline.com
	This is also the contact for MedEconomics and MIMS
	(prescribing information with excellent tables to
	compare drugs)
Pulse (newspaper)	CMP Information Ltd, City Reach,
	5 Greenwhich View Place, Millharbour,
	London E14 9NN
	Tel: 020 7861 6483
Health and Ageing	Medicom(UK) Ltd, Churston House,
	Portsmouth Road, Esher,
	Surrey KT10 9AD
	Tel: 01372 471671
Geriatric Medicine	Medpress (a division of Inside Communications Media Ltd),
	Isis Building, Thames Key,
	193 Marsh Wall, London E14 9SG
	Tel: 020 7772 8300

GP registrar money issues

Salary

This is paid by the practice (which is reimbursed by the primary care trust). It includes a car allowance.

Mileage

Mileage for visits can be claimed back from the primary care trust. This does not include mileage to work (unless there is a visit on the way).

Mileage for visits is also tax deductible. If you fill in a tax return you will have to declare the money you are reimbursed.

Defence union

This is reimbursed by the primary care trust. Usually the practice manager claims this back for you. If it is not reimbursed it is a tax-deductible expense.

Relocation allowance, telephone rental and installation can be applied for

Expenses that will probably be tax deductible

- *Professional subscriptions*: GMC, BMJ, DRCOG, DFFP, defence union, etc.
- *Mileage*: for visits, not to and from work. If you are working as a locum, all mileage is tax deductible because you are working from home.
- *Office at home*: running costs, rates, electricity, gas, etc., are worked out as a proportion, depending on the number of rooms in your house/square footage.
- *Computer*: if you use it for work.
- *Stationery*: used for work (e.g. paper, envelopes, stamps/postage, acetates).
- *MRCGP exam fees*: this is necessary if you want to be involved in training.
- *Courses*: if you pay for them (if you are reimbursed you must declare this).
- *Telephone expenses*: if you use your home telephone for work, ensure that you get an itemised bill so that you are able to calculate the correct amount. Alternatively, your accountant may use estimates.
- *Video tapes*: the videos for summative assessment and the MRCGP; you are unlikely to be able to justify the purchase of video equipment as this should be supplied by your training practice. The fees for sending things recorded delivery, etc., are also tax deductible.
- *Internet links from home.*
- *Miscellaneous*: digital camera if used for work purposes/teaching/publications (if it is also used at home, then a proportion of the cost should be calculated); any books and equipment necessary for your job.

Keep up-to-date records (ideally a spreadsheet) of all incoming and outgoings.

Speak to your accountant or to the business advisers at the Inland Revenue, as you are self-employed as a GP. The latter are an excellent source of information and will help you with your tax return if needed, but it is prudent to remember who they work for!

Remember that you will have to declare all incoming monies (e.g. cremations fees, DS1500s, etc.) from private work. Even if you have not filled in a tax return while doing your hospital jobs, you could still be investigated, and this is especially likely if your first tax return is as a GP. Get used to doing them early when the figures are easier!

Always keep all of your receipts.

Self-employment as a GP/locum

This follows on from the registrar issues. Good records are essential, and outgoings that are tax deductible are similar.

Because GPs provide a service (rather than receiving a contract of service as in other NHS professions), we have a self-employed, independent contractor status.

Once you have qualified as a GP you need to register yourself as being self-employed with the Inland Revenue. If you do not register within 3 months of starting work, you will probably be fined.

You will find some information as well as a selection of relevant publications at www.inlandrevenue.gov.uk, and the helpline number for the newly self-employed is: 08459 154 515 (this is to register; alternatively you can complete form CWF1).

By registering as self-employed you will pay Class 2 National Insurance (NI). At the end of the tax year, when you send in your self-assessment tax form, the amount of NI contributions you owe will be calculated. This is then payable as Class 4 NI at the same time as you pay your income tax bill.

You also need to ensure that you are registered with a primary care trust on their supplementary list.

Applying for locum jobs

- Negotiate pay before doing a job. Ask around to find out what other people are charging.

- Negotiate what work is to be done (length of surgery, number of appointments, visits, etc.).

- Once the job is complete, or on a weekly/monthly basis, invoice the practice:
  - if you do not do this, you are unlikely to get paid
  - if you take the invoice with you on your final day, it saves on postage, your records will be up to date, and there is less chance of forgetting what you have claimed for.

- Locums can now contribute to the superannuation scheme. Your primary care trust will have the relevant information. If you ask them, they will send you the forms that you will need the practice to complete to prove what your earnings have been. Information is also available from the NHS Pensions Agency. Tel: 01253 774774; www.NHSPA.gov.uk.

- Try to save around 40% of your income in a high-interest account for:
  - income tax
  - Class 4 National Insurance
  - superannuation
  - defence union subscriptions for next year.

Considerations when looking for a GP post

Just as when making any major decision, it is important to work out the things that are fundamentally important to you and the things you would be prepared to compromise on.

Do not feel you have to rush into anything, there are always jobs, and in the interim, locum work is not only lucrative but may help you develop your idea of how you want to work.

Below are some of the things to consider.

- Full time or part time.

- PMS or GMS practice.

- Salaried, partnership or retainer.

- Portfolio career options.

- Outside work you may want to do:
  - clinical assistant post
  - family planning
  - private health screening
  - obesity clinics
  - local medical committee
  - primary care trust work
  - post-marketing surveillance work
  - forensic work.

- If you are considering a partnership:
  - rural/inner-city location
  - where in the country
  - how many partners you want to work with
  - how many sessions you want to work
  - whether you want to be involved in training or with medical students
  - whether you want a dispensing practice
  - how involved do you want to be in antenatal care, child health, minor surgery, practice development, etc.?
  - whether other members of the primary healthcare team have a base at the practice
  - what computer system is used
  - who does the auditing
  - what role the practice nurses have (is there a nurse practitioner?)
  - what the premises are like
  - what car parking is like (small things can become very irritating)
  - how the appraisals work, who does them
  - what the local hospitals, educational meetings and outpatient waiting times are like
  - what security measures there are
  - what meetings take place (weekly business, nurse, practice, in-house educational, etc.).

- Does the practice hold social events?

- Other issues:
  - what are the local schools like?
  - what are house prices like in the area?
  - what are the road/motorway links like?

Partnership agreement

If you are a member of the BMA, request a copy of *Medical Partnership under the NHS*. This should get you orientated with regard to what issues a practice agreement should cover. You should be thinking about signing a written mutual agreement at the end of your period of mutual assessment. It is foolhardy to enter into a partnership with no written agreement in place. In such an instance this is a partnership at will, which can be brought to an end as quickly as it is formed.

It is advisable to take specialist independent legal (and accountancy) advice before signing. You need to protect yourself, no matter how well you think you know your partners.

What should it cover?

1 All parties' names and addresses.

2 Commencement date.

3 Declaration relating to termination of partnership, retirement, a party wishing to move, gross misconduct, etc.

4 Capital assets:
   − sale and purchasing of shares
   − valuation methods, especially in relation to cost rent scheme.

5 Occupation of premises by non-owning partners.

6 Expenses − individual and partnership.

7 Income − individual and partnership, especially notional/cost rent income, outside work (is it to be pooled?).

8 Schedule of profit shares from commencement date to parity.

9 Partners' obligation to each other.

10 Partnership accounts (drawings, tax reserve, year end, accountants).

11 Superannuation.

12 Holiday and study leave.

13 Sickness, maternity and paternity entitlement.

14 Effect of retirement or death − restrictive covenant.

15 Arbitration of provisions.

16 Declaration about patients.

Things to consider in detail, prior to accepting the partnership

There will be terms to negotiate, and this will involve compromise.

Commitment to the practice

- Number of sessions to be worked.

- Outside interests/work (will earnings be pooled?).

Finances

- Determine the cost of buying in and the time to parity.

- Profit share distribution.

Voting rights

Some matters should only be acted on with a unanimous agreement (e.g. appointment of a new partner).

- One vote per partner is ideal.

- Part-time partners should have equal voting power if they buy into a share of the profits but are 'jointly' liable and have the same professional interest in the business.

Maternity leave

- Currently 26 weeks, it can be claimed to cover locum costs.

- Time allowed must be fair.

- Determine what will happen to drawings and who will cover the locum costs.

- Paternity leave details are equally important.

Expulsion clauses

These may be important if you have any existing conditions. Don't presume it (e.g. lengthy incapacity, gross misconduct) will never happen to you.

Expenses

This includes all things (e.g. phones, subscriptions, courses and travel, equipment, books, etc.). There need to be explicit rules on what will be covered in the practice and what will be paid for personally.

Accounts

When considering buying into a practice, one thing it is necessary to look over and to understand (to a certain degree) is the practice accounts.

I am not an accountant and certainly make no claim to be an expert on the subject, but going through the process and having to put your name to the yearly accounts makes you learn quickly. I hope you find this Noddy-like guide a useful starting point.

In short, you are looking at four issue.

- Is the practice solvent?

- How much will you be drawing?

- Have there been any major changes from one year to the next, and why?

- Where could the practice potentially improve?

When you receive the accounts they will probably be in a summarised format (i.e. they will not include every single transaction but will have sections lumped together).

Look at the year of the accounts that you are given. Some run from 6 April to 5 April (i.e. the tax year), others run from 1 January to 31 December. It really does not matter, but do be aware that you may be looking at accounts well over 12 months old.

In the accounts you should see two columns of figures – the current year and the previous year for easy comparison. Look at each of the following.

- The layout:
  - is it a logical format?
  - is it clear where the numbers are from? If not, ask.

- How were the figures calculated?

- How did performance compare with previous years?
  - how does it compare with the national average (often represented graphically at the end of the accounts using information from *MedEconomics*)?
  - what areas can be improved?

- Are the following shown clearly:
  - value and ownership of property?
  - fixed assets (fixtures, fittings, computers, furniture, drug stock)?
  - investments and running costs?

- Is seniority pay, etc., kept personally or pooled?

- Does the practice pay for GMC, defence union and professional subscriptions, etc.?

- How much profit was made and was this shared fairly in line with the partnership agreement?

- Is there a partnership tax account?

- How much tax and National Insurance are you likely to pay?

- Is there an accountant's report (a summary of the important features of the accounts)?

Also consider the following.

- Partner's current accounts are drawn up by the accountant (i.e. not a separate account, as if each partner had their own account within the business). They are likely to include, for example, seniority pay areas where one partner may assume all responsibility, etc. It is recommended that these accounts are zeroed each year. If a substantial amount builds up the practice could go into the red if a partner were to leave and want that money reimbursed.

- Getting professional help to go through the accounts with you (a specialist in GP finance and accountancy).

- Sources of private income (insurance certificates, medicals, sick notes, etc.).

- If a practice is doing well above or below average, why is this? Remember that if fraud is committed (i.e. incorrect claims), money will have to be reimbursed to the primary care trust, and there may be criminal proceedings. In this situation, all partners are liable.

Useful websites

Royal College of General Practitioners
www.rcgp.org.uk

British Medical Association
www.bma.org.uk

General Medical Council
www.gmc_uk.org

Bandolier (useful evidence-based reviews)
www.ebandolier.com

Cochrane Library
www.cochranelibrary.com/cochrane

Centre for Evidence-based Medicine
www.cebm.net

British National Formulary
www.bnf.vhn.net

Drug Information
www.druginfozone.nhs.uk

Medicines and Healthcare Products Regulatory Agency
www.mhra.gov.uk

Prescribing database
www.emims.net

TOXOBASE
www.spib.axl.co.uk

Department of Health
www.doh.gov.uk

Health Protection Agency
www.hpa.org.uk

GP Website Database
www.gpwebsites.net

Patient Group Directives
www.nelm.nhs.uk/PGD

GP-UK discussion group
www.jiscmail.ac.uk/lists/gp-uk.html

NHS Information Authority
www.nhsia.nhs.uk

National electronic Library for Health
www.nelh.nhs.uk

Search engine
www.medisearch.co.uk

NHS Delivery Practice Database (interactive)
www.doh.gov.uk/learningzone/sdpinter.htm

HAZnet (Health Action Zones)
www.haznet.org.uk

National Institute for Mental Health in England
www.doh.gov.uk/mentalhealth.nimhe.htm

Index

Page numbers in *italic* refer to figures or tables.